# PCP: THE DEVIL'S DUST

Recognition, Management,
and Prevention of
Phencyclidine Abuse

**Ronald L. Linder, Ed.D.**
**with**
**Steven E. Lerner, Ph.D.**
**R. Stanley Burns, M.D.**

Wadsworth Publishing Company
Belmont, California
A Division of Wadsworth, Inc.

Continuing Education Editor: Nancy Taylor
Production Editor: Jeanne Heise
Designers: Detta Penna, Steve Renick
Copy/Developmental Editor: Robert McNally

Printed in the United States of America

1 2 3 4 5 6 7 8 9 10 — 85 84 83 82 81

**Library of Congress Cataloging in Publication Data**

Linder, Ronald L
    PCP, the Devil's dust.

    Bibliography: p.
    Includes index.
    1. Phencyclidine.    I. Lerner, Steven E., joint author.    II. Burns, Richard Stanley, 1944 – joint author.    III. Title. [DNLM: 1. Drug abuse — Prevention and control.    2. Phencyclidine. QV77.7 L744p]
    RC568.P45L56            362.2'9            80-23097
    ISBN 0-534-00954-9

*To those PCPers and their families who shared a part of their lives with us.*

# iv CONTENTS

This book is the outgrowth of seven years of research into recognizing, managing, and preventing phencyclidine (PCP) abuse. That research has uncovered a great many approaches to the problem, some of them appropriate, but some of them clearly risky for PCP abusers (PCPers) or human service providers. Our concern for this problem and the many requests for information about PCP prompted us to write this book.

That decision involved us deeply in the dilemma faced by everyone involved professionally with drug abuse. Historically, the hazards of psychoactive drugs have been overstated and sensationalized. We are all familiar with the official horror stories of the 1930s about the "killerweed" marijuana and with the claims by liquor industry lobbyists that marijuana was the first step to heroin addiction. Nonsense of the same sort was repeated when LSD first appeared on the street, when amphetamines became common, when cocaine turned into a popular recreational chemical for the well-to-do. Obviously, we do not want to fall into the same trap of crying wolf when a lesser alarm would do.

The best way to determine the danger posed by an illicit drug is systematic research on its effects in laboratory animals and human volunteers. Such research, limited as it is, has helped us assess the true dangers of marijuana, LSD, amphetamines, and cocaine. Unfortunately, no such research is yet available for PCP, and it may appear that we are stating the dangers the drug poses before they are known or substantiated. We admit this problem, but we contend that PCP differs distinctly from the other abused drugs and that, despite the absence of systematic research, the evidence of risk is overwhelming. We have lived through the marijuana, LSD, and amphetamine movements, and we are convinced that PCP is a drug of a different and far more dangerous order.

Our research into PCP started in 1974, when R. Stanley Burns and Steven E. Lerner were working on a federally funded research team attempting to develop new treatment techniques for multiple-drug abusers. They first met PCPers while providing medical assistance during rock music concerts and later discovered that many drug abusers had used PCP regularly for as long as six years.

This discovery led them to try to assess the extent of the PCP problem by surveying local coroners. Their findings revealed fifteen deaths attributed to PCP between 1970 and 1975. "In all cases analysis of body fluids for toxicology showed the presence of phencyclidine and the absence of any other chemical agent" (1). Burns and Lerner decided to extend their inquiry by comprehensively examining a small group of chronic PCPers. Beginning with physical and neurological examinations, including chemical analyses of body fluids as well as of the actual street drugs being used, and personal histories of the PCPers, Burns and Lerner extended their work into the psychosocial implications of PCP abuse (2). A cursory survey of local police and emergency room records turned up over 1000 cases related to PCP abuse, indicating that the problem was far more extensive than anyone had anticipated. Burns and Lerner shared their interest in and concern about PCP abuse with the medical community through a series of articles that identified patterns of use, states of intoxication, social impacts, and preliminary guidelines for recognition and treatment (1– 7). The response of poison control and drug information centers to these early publications indicated clearly that PCP was becoming a new national drug problem.

As the need for professional information and advice about the drug increased, Ronald L. Linder joined the group in 1976. Our findings have been presented at National Drug Abuse Conferences, the Thirty-Eighth Annual Scientific Meeting of the National Academy of Sciences, the Sixth World Congress of Psychiatry, a special PCP conference sponsored by the National Institute on Drug Abuse, and the joint Senate hearings on phencyclidine of the Sixty-Fifth Congress of the United States. Our work has received public exposure from numerous appearances on such national television programs as "60 Minutes" and from feature articles in popular magazines.

This book is based on our study of over 2000 PCP abusers, extensive court work, and training activities throughout the United States and abroad. It culminates our work to the present and examines PCP abuse from every perspective. Chapter 1, "Defining the PCP Problem," discusses the nature of PCP, its development and multiple identities, the extent of its abuse, and efforts to control it. Chapter 2, "The Experience and Effects of PCP Abuse," focuses on the pharmacological novelty of PCP, the patterns of usage, the PCP experience, its effects on the brain and sexual functioning, its impact on the community, and common questions about PCP. Chapter 3, "Recognizing the PCPer," discusses the forms and methods of use of PCP and the techniques for managing PCPers. Chapter 4, "Managing the PCPer," is devoted primarily to guidelines for those working in law enforcement, emergency medicine, community drug treatment, and mental health. Legal issues related to PCP intoxication and the role of the expert witness are the major themes of Chapter 5, "Litigating the PCPer." Chapter 6, "Community Action to Stop PCP Abuse," stresses essential interactions between human service providers through network building and prevention, our best hope for the future.

## Acknowledgments

The authors wish to thank the following: Hugh Alcott, Darrel Clardy, Dick Cox, Dr. Ed Domino, Dr. Alan Done, George Ellis, Jr., Dr. Dick Garey, Dr. Don Green, Michael Guy, Bob Hussey, Catherine Kallick Linder, Ruth Linstrom, Mary Tuma McAdams, Don McInnis, Barbara Menz, Metro Drug Awareness, Dave and Debbie Naishtut, Dr. Cindy Naragon, PharmChem Laboratories, Gene Rudolph, Michael D. Sher, Peg Weiser, Ray Wells.

# PART I

THE PCP
PROBLEM

# CHAPTER 1                 1

DEFINING
THE PCP
PROBLEM

**2**

What PCP is depends on who you ask. Some users describe the PCP experience as a combination of sniffing glue and taking LSD; others say it is a mix of "heaven and hell." To the researcher, PCP represents a new class of drugs with effects unlike those of any previously abused drug. For those in the criminal justice system, PCP has opened a Pandora's box of issues and problems for which traditional responses are inappropriate. The social worker finds that PCPers are among the most difficult clients to reintegrate into the community. The schoolteacher finds PCP a disruption in the classroom and another barrier to learning. Medical and mental health professionals have been confused by the masquerading symptoms of PCP patients and have mistakenly treated them with inappropriate medication, exploratory surgery, and electroconvulsive therapy (1–3).

Whatever perspective one takes, PCP is a major drug problem. The figure below represents a breakdown of drug-related admissions to county-operated emergency rooms in Los Angeles, California, in 1978. Approximately 18 percent of all drug-related admissions (7470) were for PCP or PCP in combination with other drugs (4,5). This is only an average figure. In one of the larger

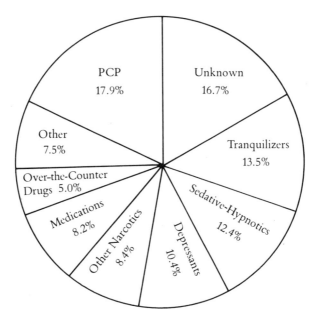

hospitals, half of all drug-related admissions were for PCP. And the problem is getting worse. PCP-related admissions in Los Angeles increased to 22.5 percent during the first half of 1979 (5), a trend possibly true for major cities throughout the United States.

**3**

## How the PCP Problem Developed

Chemically, PCP is 1-(1-phencyclohexyl) piperidine hydrochloride, the prototype of the phencyclidines. This family of chemicals contains some thirty similar compounds, called analogs, and researchers estimate that there may be as many as 120 variations of PCP (6,7)

PCP started out as a medical compound with considerable promise, but adverse side effects prevented its adoption for general use (8–10). Like many other drugs proven medically unacceptable, PCP then made its way onto the street.

### PCP in Medicine

The groundwork for synthesizing PCP was laid in 1926, but it was not until 1956 that studies of the drug in monkeys found it to be a potent analgesic and anesthetic. PCP works differently from other anesthetics, increasing rather than depressing respiration, heart rate, and blood pressure. This effect interested researchers who wanted an anesthetic that could be used on patients endangered by the depressed heart rate and blood pressure induced by other anesthetics. In 1957 initial clinical studies were carried out to determine whether PCP could be used routinely as an effective and safe general anesthetic. PCP proved a good anesthetic, but patients given the drug often suffered from confusion and excitement during recovery, a fact that dampened medical enthusiasm for the drug. Because of PCP's mind-altering characteristics, British psychiatrists in the early 1960s tried the drug experimentally on their patients in psychotherapy.

**4**

In 1963 PCP was released for further testing by Parke–Davis and Company as Sernyl. Sernyl was found to be effective as an anesthetic for major surgery at a dose of 20 milligrams (mg) injected intravenously. The drug was also used to control pain in severely burned children.

Children, it appeared, were less prone to experience adverse side effects. Adult patients compared the initial sensations of Sernyl to being drunk, sometimes accompanied by dizziness or sleep. "My legs are a mile away. . . . I feel huge and spongy one moment and tiny the next. . . . Everyone's voice is really loud. . . . This is like being in a submarine. . . . I'm floating. . . . I am now two people watching each other. . . . I'm scared. I feel like I'm going to die" were typical responses of patients who received the drug (11,12). Further administration of the drug prompted various reactions: head movements, grimacing, flailing of the arms, stiffening of the legs, shouting, muscle tension, nausea and vomiting, persistent confusion, mood changes, and convulsions (from large doses). Many patients later reported that their experiences were frightening and unpleasant. Some suffered from anxiety and insomnia for as long as five days.

Older patients coming out of an anesthetic dose of Sernyl frequently reported they felt several years younger, as though they had been "born again." Both young and middle-aged patients tended to differ only by sex in their recovery. Males were apt to be aggressive and violent, requiring constant supervision for several hours. Females generally appeared happily intoxicated, sometimes giggling and laughing, and usually required no special care.

Upon recovery, older patients tended not to remember anything that happened for up to five hours after receiving Sernyl. Younger patients reported more hallucinations even though they could not recall surgery or returning to their hospital room. Children often described their experiences as being in "Alice's wonderland." Investigators found that the altered state of consciousness produced by PCP is "much closer to schizophrenia than that produced by LSD" (13).

Some patients who experienced adverse side effects from PCP asked never to be given the drug again. For example, a middle-aged male who thought he was dying throughout a minor surgical procedure under PCP anesthesia said, "The experience was the worst in my life." Evidence was mounting that PCP's side effects were unpredictable, yet, undeniably, the drug was an effective anesthetic. **5** A debate rose between PCP's defenders and its detractors. The following two letters from the January 1963 *Anesthesia* represent the opposing sides (14,15).

Sir,

I was amazed to see two articles in the October issue of *Anesthesia* on phencyclidine. I thought this drug had been respectably buried two or three years ago.

Dr. Riddoch has used this drug in Aberdeen on children, and comes to the conclusion that it produced a number of serious side effects and was not worth further investigation . . . and I for one will agree with her conclusions. I am, however, disturbed by the article by Dr. Camilleri. He states that only three patients had any dreams or hallucinations, that they lasted for a maximum of three to four hours and were completely forgotten the next day. . . . He gives the further impression that this is a useful drug and its further investigation is desirable.

Some time ago one of my juniors, albeit an experienced anesthetist, gave this drug to a patient for a manipulation of shoulder at one of our outlying hospitals. He came back and told me how well it had worked and how pleased everyone was with its effect. Later in the week I met the patient, who happened to be a male nurse, and when he was preparing to move a patient whom I had just anaesthetised, he told me in rather an agitated manner that he had had "a bad experience" with a new drug. On being asked a few simple questions about this, he poured forth quite a torrent of words: He had never felt so terrible in his life. He didn't know what to do with himself and thought "he was going round the bend." Now he knew what his own patients felt like. If he ever had another operation, he would rather have it with no anesthetic at all than live through this experience again.

I had known this man for some years and always looked upon him as a steady, not easily agitated type, and although he was obviously relieved when I assured him that such drug-induced hallucinations could not recur once the drug had been eliminated, it was one or two weeks before he regained his equilibrium.

The risk of administering such a drug to a patient should not be taken, even if the chances of such a result are only one in 10,000, and to administer it to women who can be subject to puerperal [postpartum] psychosis from no known cause strikes me as highly dangerous.

I feel very strongly on this matter and as it may be some time before you are able to publish this letter, I propose to send a copy to the manufacturers, and suggest that they withdraw the drug from further trial.

Yours faithfully,
F.F. Waddy
General Hospital
Northampton

**6**

Sir,

Dr. F. F. Waddy kindly supplied us with a draft of his letter dated 31 October, addressed to yourself.

His description of the male nurse's experience is typical of many reports we received at that time (two or three years ago). The fact that phencyclidine is still undergoing active clinical trial might have suggested to Dr. Waddy that this is no longer true. His male nurse would no doubt react in the same way today as he did then, but he would not now be anesthetised with this new drug.

The purpose of clinical trials is to obtain information, and in the course of four years a great deal of information has been obtained about phencyclidine. A brief summary of some of the more important facts follows:

1. Phencyclidine is an unsuitable anesthetic agent for young and middle-aged adults — especially adults. Subjects in these age groups are especially prone to develop hallucinations, which though usually pleasant, are occasionally excessively objectionable.

2. In old people (over sixty-five) these undesirable effects are exceedingly uncommon if they occur at all.

3. In small children (under six) the drug is also satisfactory as an anesthetic. [However] it cannot be considered as a sedative, hypnotic, or tranquilizer. Only in frail old people should phencyclidine be used as, or instead of, premedication [before anesthesia].

4. The very old and the very young not only tolerate phencyclidine anesthesia well, but derive the greatest advantage from its unique properties, namely, the absence of respiratory or cardiovascular depression and the safety of using the drug shortly after a meal.

5. Evidence is accumulating, though as yet by no measure complete, that parturient [in labor or giving birth] women tolerate phencyclidine better than nonpregnant women of the same age. In a recent series of 561 cases anesthetised with phencyclidine, including 377 anesthetics given for obstetrical indications, hallucination occurred on sixteen occasions. It is not stated what proportion of these were objectionable. Against this occasional occurrence of hallucinations must be set the extreme safety of the drug. Though well over 3000 subjects have now been anesthetised with phencyclidine, many of them more than once, in no case has any permanent harmful effect been attributed to the drug, in spite of the fact that large overdoses have occasionally been inadvertently given. Of what other agent in an anesthetist's armamentarium could the same be said?

> Yours faithfully,
> J. A. L. Gorringe,
> Director
> Department of Clinical
> Investigation
> Parke-Davis and Company

All in all, over 1500 patients in the United States were given phencyclidine between 1958 and 1967. Of the 1200 obstetrical and surgi-

cal patients receiving a single dose of PCP, no cases of persistent or
repeated psychosis resulting from the drug were reported. In addition, 200 psychiatric patients were given subanesthetic doses, and
only 6 suffered intensified psychological problems — suggesting
that the "set," the "setting," and the dose are critical factors affecting the patient's reaction to the drug.

Yet, even though PCP's adverse effects appeared transient, they
were common enough and unpleasant enough that even those who
had advocated the drug turned against it. In January 1965 Parke-
Davis and Company requested the Food and Drug Administration
to withdraw phencyclidine from use on humans.

PCP can still be had in certain pharmaceutical applications,
however. Renamed *Sernylan,* PCP was available commercially as a
veterinary drug until 1979. A phencyclidine derivative sold commercially as Ketamine produces the same anesthetic effects as PCP
but with fewer adverse reactions. It is still used on humans. Also,
the Food and Drug Administration has been requested to approve
the marketing of a combination of Ketamine and Valium. Valium is
used to control the side effects of the Ketamine, making the drug
medically more useful. Ironically, it also increases the drug's potential for abuse.


## PCP on the Street


About the same time that phencyclidine under a new trade name
became a veterinary drug, it appeared on the streets of San Francisco. There it received the name PCP for *PeaCe Pill,* because the
drug was reputed to give the illusion of everlasting peace. PCP did
not live up to its name. The inexperienced users of the new drug
culture were unprepared for PCP's bizarre effects, and they
criticized the substance in much the same terms as clinical patients
before them. Within a year, PCP had vanished from the Haight-
Ashbury, but PCP reappeared as "hog" in New York City. On the
East Coast PCP met the same run of bad reviews as on the West
Coast, and it was soon written off as a "bummer" drug.

In the early 1970s, however, PCP staged a comeback. PCP was
usually mixed with other drugs, mostly LSD at first, then with an
unprecedented host of other common psychoactive agents spanning
the spectrum from marijuana to heroin. Times had changed. The

same bizarre effects that had caused earlier drug users to dismiss the drug as dangerous now attracted a new generation of experimenters. Unfortunately, these new users didn't stop at experimenting on themselves. Like missionaries, they sought to convert others through the baptism of PCP intoxication, which became the cement of their social relationships. "When you run on dust," the saying went, "it runs you. Every waking moment you spend talking, hustling, or using" (16).

All evidence (PCP deaths, emergency room contacts, and police arrests) indicated that by 1974 Alameda County, California — an urban area including Berkeley and Oakland — had become the center of the new PCP culture. The drug became commonplace. For example, of eighty-six urine samples taken from drivers assumed to be under the influence of alcohol, forty-eight tested positive for PCP exclusively and six for PCP in combination with other drugs (17,18). Parents, social workers, teachers, and police officers found themselves confronting seemingly unexplained cases of memory loss, speech problems, severe personality and mood changes, thought disorders, anxiety, depression, and suicidal behavior. Also, PCP was implicated in a dramatic number of deaths by drowning, fire, falls, vehicle accidents, homicide, suicide, and overdose (19).

Alameda County was only the beginning. As with other street drugs, a ripple effect spread PCP to the East Coast and then to other cities. By 1977 major-city newspapers and national newsmagazines were discussing PCP abuse. Local and national television also recognized the problem in news coverage, a "60 Minutes" segment entitled "Angel Dust/PCP," and several episodes in prime-time series about the drug. The obvious had become apparent: PCP was, and is, a major drug problem.

## PCP's Many Identities

Over a period of seven years we have attempted to identify different names used for PCP. These names reflect the reports of poison control and drug information centers, street drug analysis programs,

law enforcement agencies, and extensive personal communications **9**
with the human service providers we have trained. As the list
shows, the phencyclidines have many common street names. Some
of the names provide descriptive evidence of the many forms the
drug may take. For example, in southern California, lovely is PCP
and marijuana in combination. Peanut butter, in New Orleans, is
PCP added to actual peanut butter. In Chicago, rocket fuel is PCP
and cocaine. The names of other drugs in italic print have been used
to market PCP. The vast majority of these preparations are combinations of PCP and other drugs, occasionally the actual drug
named.

| | | |
|---|---|---|
| Ace | D | Herms |
| Ad | Detroit pink | Hog |
| Amoeba | Devil's dust | Horse tranquilizer |
| *Amphetamine* | Dipper | Jet fuel |
| Animal | *DMT* | Juice |
| Animal tranquilizer | DOA | K |
| Angel dust | Dog | K–Blast |
| Angel hair | Double dipper | Kaps |
| Angel mist | Dummy dust | *Ketamine* |
| Aurora borealis | Dust | Killerweed |
| *Belladonna* | Dust joint | KJ crystal |
| Black whack | Elephant | Kools |
| Busy bee |    tranquilizer | KW |
| Cadillac | Embalming fluid | Lemmon 714 |
| *Cannabinol* | Energizer | Lenos |
| Cigarrode cristal | Erth | Live ones |
| CJ | Flakes | Lovely |
| *Cocaine* | Fuel | *LSD* |
| Coke | Goon | Magic |
| Columbo | Goon dust | Magic dust |
| Cozmos | Gorilla Tab | *MDA* |
| Cristal | Green | Mean green |
| Crystal | Green tea | *Mescaline* |
| Crystal points | *Hashish* | Mintweed |
| Crystal T | Heaven and Hell | Mist |
| Cyclones | *Heroin* | Monkey dust |

| | | |
|---|---|---|
| More | *Psilocybin* | Surfer |
| New magic | Puffy | Synthetic cocaine |
| Niebla | *Quaalude* | T |
| Orange crystal | Rocket fuel | TAC |
| Ozone | Scaffle | Tea |
| Parsley | Sheets | *THC* |
| PAZ | Sherms | TIC |
| *PCP* | Smoking | Trank |
| PCPA | Snorts | TT-1 |
| Peace | Soma | TT-2 |
| PeaCe Pill | Spores | TT-3 |
| Peaceweed | Star dust | Water |
| Peanut butter | Stick | Weed |
| Peter Pan | *STP* | Whack wack |
| *Peyote* | Super | White powder |
| Pig killer | Super | Wobble weed |
| Polvo | Super grass | Worm |
| Polvo de angel | Super joint | Yellow fever |
| Polvo de | Super kools | Zombie weed |
|     estrellas | Super weed | Zoom |

PCP goes by more names and comes in more colors than all other street drugs combined. Its actual colors are various shades of white. Other colors are usually specific to the locale. Dealers report that if business is slow, they change the color of their product and sell it by a different name — often to counter adverse publicity on a bad batch of local PCP.

Illicitly made PCP has continuously changed in physical form. It has appeared on the streets as a powder, tablet or capsule, leaf mixture, liquid, and crystal or granule, with the last of these the most common. When found on parsley, mint, oregano, tobacco, or other leaves, PCP is usually in the form of a "joint" (20).

PCP's purity also varies — by batch, source, locale, and form. The crystalline or granular powder, sold as crystal or angel dust, ranges from 50 to 100 percent pure PCP. Purchased by most other names, it is from 10 to 30 percent pure. Tablets usually contain from 2 to 6 milligrams (mg) of PCP. Leaf mixtures have been found to contain on the average 1 to 8 mg. Nevertheless, samples have been found containing as much as 150 mg of PCP (21,22). Some of the street samples analyzed for PCP contain many other drugs —

barbiturates, cocaine, ethyl alcohol, heroin, LSD, mescaline, **11**
methadone, procaine, and Quaalude (20). As many as five other
drugs have been detected in samples alleged to be pure PCP.

As PCP has become more popular, it has appeared on the street
mixed with several of its analogs (23). PCE (N-ethyl-1-
phenylcyclohexylamine) was first detected in California in 1970 and
then in Illinois in 1973. Since that time, it has appeared in such states
as Louisiana, Oklahoma, Indiana, Alabama, Florida, Georgia, and
Kansas. PCPY [1-(1-phenycyclohexyl) pyrrolidine] was first identified in Maryland in 1974 and has since appeared in California,
Florida, Nevada, New Jersey, and New York. TCP [1-
(1-(2-thienyl) cyclohexyl) piperidine] was first seen in California
and later in Hawaii, Washington, and Oregon. Recently, Ketamine
and PCPY have been popular, probably because of their supposed
aphrodisiac effects on women.

Most likely the analogs have become more common in part because more underground laboratories are in the business of making
PCP. Also, some underground chemists have made the analogs
either because they are more potent than prototypical PCP or because they are not yet illegal. PCE, for example, was originally not
a controlled substance. An underground maker in the South produced 100 pounds of PCE and distributed it free, an act the police
were legally powerless to stop.

This loophole in the law has been partly patched. As of this date,
the following PCP analogs are under federal control, with others
pending:

- TCP or 1-(1-(2-thienyl) cyclohexyl) piperidine hydrochloride
- PCE or N-ethyl-1-phenylcyclohexylamine hydrochloride
- PCPY or 1-(1-phenylcyclohexyl) pyrrolidine hydrochloride
- PCC or 1-piperdinocyclohexanecarbonitrile
- PCP or phencyclidine hydrochloride
- 1-phenylcyclohexylamine hydrochloride

Adding to the confusion complicating the PCP picture, PCP has
commonly been used to adulterate other drugs. A laboratory in
California made the following typical findings (24):

| Alleged Substance | Actual Substance | Appearance |
| --- | --- | --- |
| THC | PCP | Tan powder |
| LSD | PCP | Lavender tablet |
| Mescaline | PCP + LSD | Red–brown tablet |
| Cocaine | PCP + PCC + lactose | White powder |
| Psilocybin | PCP + LSD | Mushroom pieces |
| Synthetic Cocaine | Ketamine | Green plant material |

Of the different names used for PCP, THC, the active ingredient in marijuana, was the most common. In retrospect, the "masquerade" of PCP as THC was an ingenious conspiracy that allowed the marketing of a new, easily made, and highly profitable drug with a bad reputation in the guise of a widely accepted and supposedly safe substance. Writers in the underground press picked up signs that something was amiss and published warnings that buyers were getting "burned" and that THC does not remain stable except at very low temperatures. Younger drug users dismissed these warnings as so much older-generation nay-saying and used the purported THC anyway. They became the primary consumers of PCP and subsequently came to prefer it. Masquerade PCP, perhaps the greatest hoax in the history of illicit drug abuse, was here to stay.

Despite the common association of the two drugs, PCP was seldom mixed with marijuana in the early 1970s, since THC is alleged to increase its potency, and since other leaf materials were cheaper and legal to possess. In the laboratory samples of PCP adulterations cited above, PCP was actually combined with marijuana in only 2 of 317 street drug samples — even though it was commonly said to be THC (21). By 1979, however, pushers had resorted to mixing PCP with marijuana as a marketing strategy. The mixture appears to have grown popular, probably because of the mistaken ideas that anything that can be smoked is safe and that PCP dosage is best controlled by smoking. Probably PCP is becoming more popular among marijuana users.

The PCP masquerade continues today. For example, recent street samples from California, Ohio, and Florida that appeared to be pharmaceutical Quaalude proved upon analysis to be PCP alone (25,26). However, masquerade PCP seems less important these days. As the drug has grown more popular under its real identity, dealers have sold it by its appropriate name, color, and form. Thus **13** a southern California street-drug information program reports that since 1975 adulteration of PCP with other drugs has dropped from 60 percent to 25 percent of all samples analyzed. The masquerade continues, though. In April 1980 methamphetamine being sold as crystal was confusing PCPers in southern California, who had used the same name for PCP for ten years.

## The Extent of PCP Abuse

When PCP reappeared on the streets in the early 1970s, it took everyone by surprise. Police officers, who often were the first professionals to have to deal with PCP's bizarre effects on behavior, found themselves confronting everything from a San Jose man who tore his eyes out to a Detroit youth with a baseball bat calling the arresting officer a giant bat, yet they had no idea what was causing these incredible episodes. Medical personnel were in a similar quandary. Faced with masquerade PCP, a confusing crowd of street names, and a puzzling array of unpredictable symptoms, they often misdiagnosed PCP intoxication and mistakenly treated PCPers for everything from meningitis to schizophrenia.

These confusions and problems greatly complicate a clear understanding of the extent of PCP abuse. Since users often do not know exactly what they have taken, the only certain test for PCP is toxicological analysis of body fluids or tissues. In the absence of such definite evidence, we can only examine sources of suggestive information (e.g., drug-related deaths, nonfatal drug abuse emergencies, and drug law violation arrests) to come up with a crude sense of how widespread PCP abuse is (7).

## Statistical Sources

PharmChem Laboratories of Menlo Park, California, analyzes street drug samples submitted by users and others, and its reports offer an indication of the extent of PCP abuse. PharmChem reports between 1972 and August 1980 indicate the spread of PCP use across the country. In 1972 PCP was detected in drug samples from five states. This figure rose to seventeen states in 1973, twenty-one in 1974, twenty-two in 1975, twenty-four in 1976, and twenty-nine in 1977. Over these years, PCP has appeared in drug samples from a total of forty-six of the fifty states. PCP can be found nearly everywhere in the country.

Curiously, the number of PCP samples fell off to thirteen states in 1978 and fourteen in 1979. For the first eight months of 1980, samples containing the phencyclidines were received from Arizona, California, Connecticut, Illinois, Massachusetts, New York, and Oregon. This does not mean that PCP has suddenly become less common — indeed, the evidence is quite the opposite. More likely, PCP users have grown sophisticated about what they are taking and no longer need to send it out for analysis.

The Drug Abuse Warning Network (DAWN) is a federally funded program aimed at detecting changes in drug-abuse patterns from data provided by emergency rooms and medical examiners. DAWN reported 22 PCP-related deaths in the United States in 1975, 35 in 1977, and 124 in 1978 (27). These figures are rough and almost certainly understated. For example, the Los Angeles coroner's office verified 111 PCP deaths in that city alone and the state of Virginia documented 40 PCP fatalities in 1978, making the phencyclidines second only to alcohol as the cause of death by drugs.

Another federal system, the Client Oriented Data Acquisition Process (CODAP), reports the drugs used by patients in federal drug abuse treatment and rehabilitation programs. However, CODAP's data tell us little about PCP abuse, because the majority of drug abuse treatment programs receive no federal funds and because CODAP misclassified PCP as a hallucinogen until March 1979.

The National Youth Polydrug Study, conducted from September 1976 to February 1977, attempted to determine the extent of PCP abuse by studying 2750 young people of twelve to eighteen years of age selected from 97 of about 350 drug treatment programs in thirty-nine states. Roughly 31 percent of the subjects had used PCP. Of these, 67 percent reported using PCP at least once a week for no less than a month. The average age of first use was 14.6 years, and by 14.8 years many continued to use the drug repeatedly (20,28).

Another study, conducted in 1978, took a random sample of 35,317 students from the nearly 2 million enrolled in grades seven to twelve in

New York State. An estimated 14 percent (257,000) of the entire popu- **15**
lation had used PCP at least once. Use increased by grade:

| Grade | Students Using PCP at Least Once | |
|---|---|---|
| 7 | 16,000 | (5.2%) |
| 8 | 27,000 | (9.2%) |
| 9 | 48,000 | (14.9%) |
| 10 | 59,000 | (17.9%) |
| 11 | 56,000 | (20.4%) |
| 12 | 51,000 | (21.6%) |

Eleven thousand students claimed they had used PCP at least ten
times within the past thirty days. Forty-six percent of the students
reported their first PCP experience in 1977 or 1978, indicating that
the PCP problem has arisen recently and rapidly (29).

In July 1979, the National Institute on Drug Abuse (NIDA)
added PCP separately to its sampling instrument. Survey results
indicated that almost 13 percent of the sample had used PCP (30).

National Student Drug Use 1979 (N=15,500)

| | % Ever Used |
|---|---|
| Alcohol | 93.0 |
| Cigarettes | 74.0 |
| Marijuana | 60.4 |
| Stimulants | 24.2 |
| Tranquilizers | 16.3 |
| Cocaine | 15.4 |
| Sedatives | 14.6 |
| Hallucinogens | 14.1 |
| PCP | 12.8 |
| Inhalants | 12.7 |
| Heroin and other opiates | 11.2 |

Officials estimate that 7 million Americans have tried PCP.

The criminal justice system also provides suggestive evidence about the extent of PCP abuse. Arrests for PCP violations made by the Los Angeles County Sheriff's Department and the Los Angeles Police Department totaled 320 in 1975, 1260 in 1976, 6060 in 1977, 8564 in 1978, and 8152 in 1979.

A three-month study in early 1979 of 712 parolees in southern California disclosed that 13 percent of randomly collected urine samples tested positive for PCP. Among the 91 parolees with PCP in their urine, one-third had been convicted of violent crime. Collectively, among the 2000 parolees randomly screened for drugs during 1979, PCP use was the most prevalent violation (31).

**Percentage of Positive Urines**

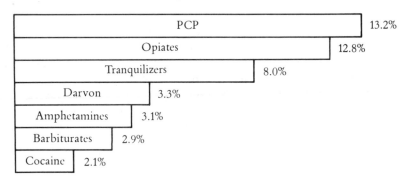

PCP has even invaded the military. No figures are available, but military officials have expressed concern over PCP abuse by duty personnel. These reports raise the specter of PCPers with access to weapon systems and of armed forces unable to meet their defense obligations because of the effects of PCP.

## The Underground PCP Movement

PCP is easy to make. Cookbook recipes have been published in the underground press, and would-be manufacturers need little more than a basic knowledge of chemistry or cookery, some easily obtained equipment, and less than $100 worth of chemicals. PCP can be supplied easily, but for drug makers to turn the high profits their trade offers, there must be a demand for their wares. Thus the size of the underground PCP manufacturing operations suggests just **17** how big the PCP problem is.

PCP laboratories have been seized all over the country. Some are small operations, obviously aimed at nothing more ambitious than a neighborhood market, but others are much bigger. A commercial chemist in Maryland was arrested in 1974 while making ninety pounds of PCP. He was a very small fish. In 1979, 900 pounds of PCP were confiscated in a clandestine laboratory in Los Angeles, and almost 1000 pounds were recovered in Livingston, Louisiana, in 1978 (23). The dollar values of these seizures can be staggering. A graduate student in Stockton, California, used a university laboratory to make liquid PCP worth $850,000 on the street. A laboratory in an automobile repair shop in Deerfield Beach, Florida, had enough ingredients on hand to produce $39 million worth of PCP. And four private homes in northern Virginia, two in Colorado, and one in Los Angeles were manufacturing sites for a ring of eight PCP makers, who were indicted for conspiring to make PCP valued at up to $40 million.

Of course, few PCP operations are actually seized. It is estimated that in Los Angeles alone fifty individuals and groups are mass-producing PCP and that literally hundreds of others are in the business on a smaller scale (23).

An Impression

There are few hard data on the extent of PCP abuse. Still, the limited statistical evidence and the record of police actions indicate clearly that PCP has become a commonplace and widespread drug problem.

## Efforts to Eradicate PCP Abuse

When PCP hit the streets in 1967 and 1968, the federal government responded by putting PCP on the schedule of controlled drugs in 1970. This provided a statute for prosecuting individuals for posses-

**18**

sing or selling the drug, but it also stopped all ongoing clinical research into the pharmacology of PCP and limited and discouraged any future research. As a result, basic pharmacological knowledge was lacking when the PCP epidemic began, making recognition of acute PCP intoxication and rational management and treatment impossible.

The federal government's response to PCP abuse has been ineffective (32– 34), in part because of this incomplete early research. It impressed researchers working in these early and largely unfinished projects that their subjects refused to take PCP a second time. They assumed that PCP's unpleasant side effects would prevent abuse of the drug. This attitude pervaded the federal bureaucracy, and it wasn't until media coverage like the "60 Minutes" program focused popular concern on PCP that the National Institute on Drug Abuse (NIDA) paid any attention at all to the drug. Unfortunately, NIDA has done little more than pay attention. There is still no comprehensive federal response to PCP abuse.

In the absence of a national effort, state and local agencies have taken matters into their own hands. September 1978, for example, marked the beginning of a two-year PCP Training and Prevention Program throughout California. In two years over 8000 workers in community mental health, criminal justice, drug abuse treatment, emergency medicine, recreation, and public education were trained in interdisciplinary workshops to recognize and respond appropriately to the PCP problem. This project brought together, through community linking and network building strategies, human service providers needing the knowledge and skills to recognize, manage, and prevent PCP abuse. Similar training programs, now in various stages of development, will be implemented throughout the United States during the 1980s.

## Summary

PCP is the prototype of the phencyclidines, a family of at least thirty analogs. The substance showed medical promise as an anesthetic, but bad side effects led to withdrawal of the drug for use on humans. As a street drug, PCP was at first rejected as unpleasant, but it returned and grew increasingly popular in the 1970s.

PCP has many identities. It goes by dozens of street names and **19** comes in several forms and colors. PCP is also commonly used as a masquerade or adulterant for other drugs. Masquerade PCP is becoming less important, probably because PCP is more and more a street drug of choice. A number of PCP analogs have also appeared on the illicit market.

There is little hard evidence of the extent of PCP abuse. Studies, criminal justice statistics, and the production and profitability of underground PCP manufacturing all point to extensive and pervasive PCP abuse.

No comprehensive federal program has been developed to deal with PCP abuse. State and local agencies have turned to training programs for professionals involved with the PCP problem.

# CHAPTER 2

# THE EXPERIENCE AND EFFECTS OF PCP ABUSE

PCP is a unique drug, unlike anything we have met before. Because the problems it poses are so novel, understanding PCP abuse has forced us to go back to the basics. This chapter begins there, with a summary of how psychoactive drugs affect behavior and a discussion of where PCP fits among the other abused substances. Then we examine what we know of PCP's physical and mental effects on users and consider the costs of the drug to the community.

## Psychoactive Drugs and Behavior

Behavior, personality, values, and culture all have one common denominator — biochemistry. Altering the chemistry of the brain instantly changes how you feel, think, and behave. Drugs work by altering the chemistry of the brain. In simplified terms, drugs work because they disrupt the natural biochemical equilibrium of the body.

The brain is a complex organ whose millions of nerve cells are linked into billions of circuits by electrochemical transmissions. Altering the chemistry of the brain alters the circuitry of the brain. Chemically the brain can be programmed, deprogrammed, reprogrammed, impaired, and even destroyed.

Specialized cells on the surfaces of our bodies pick up information about our environment in forms we recognize as the senses of sight, hearing, touch, smell, and taste. For example, specialized cells on the interior rear surface, or retina, of the eyeball translate light into electrochemical signals. These signals travel along nerves into the brain, where they are sent to a particular area that decodes the information from the eye and interprets it. The transmission points along the line from sensory input to the brain's final processing are the sites of action of many psychoactive drugs. The behavior of an intoxicated user sometimes provides clues about the portion of the brain affected. For example, the drunk's slurred speech, dilated eyes, and unsteady balance indicate that alcohol affects the brain areas controlling speech, eye response, and balance.

This simple model of the effects of psychoactive drugs is greatly complicated by the fact that the unique characteristics of each individual and the social setting greatly influence the effects of a drug.

Marijuana, as one example, may produce effects ranging from elation and sexual arousal to depression and withdrawal, depending on the mood of the user and the setting in which the drug is taken.

## The Uniqueness of PCP

PCP further complicates this already complicated picture because its effects differ so profoundly from those of other known drugs. Many of the popular abused drugs fit into three basic classes: (1) uppers, which have a stimulant effect, like cocaine and amphetamines; (2) downers, which depress the body and the mind, like alcohol and barbiturates; and (3) outers, which create their own subjective reality, like LSD and mescaline. PCP's effects sometimes mimic the uppers, the downers, or the outers.

These varying effects appeared in the early animal experiments with PCP (1,2). In rodents, the drug worked like an upper yet it also caused drunkenness and uncoordination. Monkeys given large doses were first quiet and calm, then anesthetized enough to allow painless surgery. Dogs yelped and went into convulsions (3,4).

The dosage of the drug determined whether PCP acted as an upper or a downer. As dosage increased, the effects moved up a scale from excitement and agitation to ataxia (uncoordinated gait) to catalepsy (unusual posture) to anesthesia-analgesia to convulsions with respiratory depression. In addition, PCP's effects varied by species. At low doses monkeys were serene but mice were excited and agitated, and anesthesia did not appear in mice. This table shows the differences between the two groups. Humans showed

| Effects | Mice | Monkeys |
| --- | --- | --- |
| Excitement/agitation | + | − |
| Ataxia | + | + |
| Catalepsy | + | + |
| Anesthesia/Analgesia | − | + |
| Convulsions | + | + |

largely the same effects as monkeys. They were sensitive to the drug, went into a state of surgical anesthesia with a moderate dose, and at larger doses entered convulsions and respiratory depression (3).

PCP distorts reality, as the hallucinogens do, but it is not a hallucinogen. This fact was demonstrated by sensory deprivation research techniques, in which the subject is put in a situation where stimulation from sight, sound, and touch is greatly reduced. Early comparative research on psilocybin, LSD, and PCP revealed marked differences in thinking and sensory processes when body movements, environmental influences, and sensory stimulation were controlled experimentally (5). Psilocybin and LSD, both popular hallucinogens or psychedelics, severely distorted thinking and perception both during and after sensory deprivation. PCP, however, changed body image only subtly until the individual came out of the controlled environment. Seeing and moving normally brought on immediate distortions of perception, and these effects became more pronounced as sensory stimulation was increased.

Because PCP produces upper, downer, and outer effects, it can be mistaken for other drugs. However, awareness of PCP's uniqueness can decrease the chances of misdiagnosis. The following table charts the common signs of drug intoxication. The diagnostic symptoms of PCP are nystagmus (jerky eye movements) and elevated blood pressure, which do not appear together with any other drug abuse (6).

PCP appears to alter neurotransmission, the process by which one nerve cell releases a specific chemical to trigger an impulse in the next nerve cell (7). However, scientists are still far from identifying the sites or mechanism of PCP's action. We do know, however, that PCP is stored in fatty tissue, including the brain, from which it is slowly released — a finding that adds one more variable to the duration of the drug's effects (8).

## The Patterns of PCP Use

PCP use falls into four major categories, which form a developmental spectrum running from low risk to high.

## Common Signs and Symptoms of Drug Intoxication

| Signs and Symptoms | Phencyclidines | Stimulants | Hallucinogens | Sedative-Hypnotics | Narcotics |
|---|---|---|---|---|---|
| Aggressive and violent behavior | ● | ● | | | |
| Ataxia | ● | | | ● | |
| Coma | ● | | | ● | ● |
| Confusion | ● | | ● | | |
| Convulsions | ● | ● | | | |
| Drowsiness | ● | | | ● | ● |
| Hallucinations | ● | | ● | | |
| Hyperreflexia | ● | ● | | | |
| { Nystagmus | ● | | | ● | |
| { Hypertension | ● | ● | | | |
| Pupils { Dilated | | ● | ● | | |
|     { Pinpoint | | | | | ● |
| Paranoia | ● | ● | ● | | |
| Psychosis | ● | ● | ● | | |
| Respiratory depression | | | | ● | ● |
| Slurred speech | ● | | | ● | |

Most PCP experimenters do not report adverse effects, so experimental use of the drug is classified as low risk. However, some risk is present, because effects that cause long-term impairment or behavioral toxicity leading to injury or death are always possible. Repeated recreational exposure to PCP raises the risk of problems from behavioral toxicity or overdose. Probably the greatest risk to the recreational PCPer is increasing use to the chronic level. The chronic PCPer is continuously toxic because the drug tends to remain in the body for several days, increasing the chances of an unpredictable effect.

Surreptitious intoxication has caused much personal tragedy. We received this letter in January 1979, and the experiences it tells are all too common.

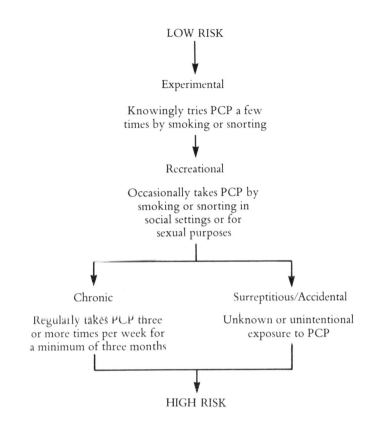

LOW RISK

Experimental

Knowingly tries PCP a few
times by smoking or snorting

Recreational

Occasionally takes PCP by
smoking or snorting in
social settings or for
sexual purposes

Chronic

Regularly takes PCP three
or more times per week for
a minimum of three months

Surreptitious/Accidental

Unknown or unintentional
exposure to PCP

HIGH RISK

Case #1116.

About six months ago I was at a party and some people gave me some
brownies that they claimed had a little grass in them. I ate a few and felt all
right until I got home. I began feeling very confused and acutely anxious. I
felt paranoid and thought I was going to die. In desperation I called the
emergency room of the hospital near here. They sent over an ambulance
since I was too confused to drive. The doctor at the hospital said I had
overdosed on PCP. By morning I was more or less better and went home. I
had never experienced anything like this before, so I was very scared. I
continued to feel dizzy and somewhat confused and depressed for the next

**26**

few weeks, and then I felt slightly better. I thought then that the effects were over, but they were not. I continued to have periods of acute anxiety every two weeks or so. It will last one to four hours and leave me feeling depressed and slightly anxious for the next few days. In some sense these attacks are a less intense version of the original incident. When I have these attacks, and for the few days afterwards, life seems hardly worth living. I was never depressed before or had any sort of similar problems. Other than these attacks everything in my life is going great, including a good job. . . .

I really hope you will know of something that might be done to help me. I have enclosed a self-addressed envelope for a reply.

P. S. My short-term memory seems also affected. I keep forgetting things I just heard or am thinking of.

The person given PCP unknowingly is at a particularly high risk. Such a person may interpret PCP's effects as an impending mental breakdown, and, because of the delusions the drug causes, it is very hard to convince the victim that the problem is PCP toxicity (drug effect), not approaching insanity.

PCP exposure may also be accidental. We have seen several cases of PCP poisoning in children.

Case#2008.

A seven-month-old baby boy was with his mother at her friend's house, where PCP was being smoked. He was discovered playing with the contents of the friend's purse, which contained a vial of PCP. Within a few minutes the infant began acting strangely. After taking him home, his mother observed unusual posturing, frothing at the mouth, and rolled back eyes. She finally took the infant to the hospital the next morning after he continued to be semiconscious. The infant was subsequently admitted to the intensive care unit for acute phencyclidine intoxication. The child's recovery was uneventful. Subsequently, the child was placed in protective custody.

In any case where accidental PCP poisoning is suspected, save some of the material and its container for analysis.

# The PCP Experience

PCP was originally written off as a "bummer" drug because of its unpleasant side effects (1–2). Thus we were surprised to discover in 1974 several groups of polydrug abusers who had been using PCP regularly for over five years. To find out why the subjective effects of PCP in patients and experimental subjects differed so much from polydrug abusers, we studied chronic users — those who had taken PCP three or more times per week for six months or longer.

Chronic PCPers reported the drug experience to be mostly pleasurable. Among one group of chronic PCPers with three to six years of regular PCP use, 80 percent considered the first drug experience desirable (9,12,13). They described their initial intoxication as "exhilarating, fun, happy, euphoric, the perfect escape, a dream world." Most experimenters compared the PCP "high" with LSD, yet they insisted it was completely different, in a class of its own. Collectively, PCP had pronounced effects on the users' thinking, time perception, sense of reality and mood. They referred to their thinking processes as "speeded up" or "wired" — "the mind going faster while time stood still." Common experiences were reported as "different, in another dimension, and seen from a new point of view. Life is dramatized into a fantasy where you don't have to dream. Your wishes are fulfilled. What you want to happen comes true." These chronic PCPers thought that everything was complete, more sensical. "The mind can focus on just one object and see beauty in the smallest thing." They described a feeling of community and oneness with others, including animals.

Many PCPers claimed that they absorbed music, felt light, and stretched space and depth from two dimensions to three. Most experienced floating sensations, and many chronic PCPers shared sensations of superhuman strength, omnipotence, and disinhibition. "God is with me and I can move mountains" is one variation of a common theme (9–13).

Religious and death experiences are relatively consistent characteristics of the chronic PCPers we have studied. Although most PCPers report intense happiness and euphoria, they also recognize the severe depression and potential for both "the heights and depths of being" while on the drug (17). Interaction with religious figures — talking with God or Christ — and the devil are not unusual. In fact, there is some evidence of a religious cult on the West Coast that uses PCP as its sacrament.

A recent psychological study of chronic PCPers supported the early accounts of the drug's subjective effects. "I feel like a rubber doll. . . . Gumbylike effects. . . . Like being drunk and loaded at the same time. . . . Everything is like a dream. . . . Things don't seem real. . . . Somewhere I've never been before. . . . No cares. . . . Spaced out. . . . Mind and body rushes" were typical descriptions given the PCP experience (17).

Acute depression is perhaps the most devastating effect of chronic PCP abuse. The following excerpts come from the suicide note of a chronic PCPer who killed himself with a PCP overdose.

To whom it may concern,
My suicide is a must. I am full of anxiety. Depression is too much. My love to Mom, Dad, Brother, and Sister. Thanks to Jane to whom I owe my availability to PCP. . . . At last I will be at peace. . . . I pray I go to Heaven and be at peace forever.

Such depression is often precipitated by an attempt to stop using the drug. As the depression becomes overwhelming, the user may try to allay the depression by taking a large amount of PCP, leading to an overdose and possible death. Some PCPers indicate that the sought-after state produced by excessive amounts is a condition of "not feeling anything," "living inside a dead body." Intermittent states of depression caused by chronic PCP abuse are like being on "an emotional roller coaster." According to one chronic PCPer, "I can be up one moment, I can be down the next, and I can be spaced out in between" (14–16).

When asked why they use PCP, respondents said, "It makes me go out and do things. . . . Music sounds better. . . . I use it for energy and for relating better to people." Others claimed, "I don't get sleepy or the munchies like I do on pot. . . . I am relaxed and have more insight. . . . I understand situations better and I'm clearer. . . . It builds my confidence to do things like meeting women. . . . It makes me more accepted. . . . It helps me just kick back and not worry." "Actually," claimed one chronic user, "the use of PCP comes down to the need or desire to escape. If you're into PCP, you're escaping." These PCP experiences evolve into a lifestyle with characteristics unlike other abused drugs.

## The PCP Lifestyle

Chronic PCPers give PCP as their first drug of choice, even though other drugs do figure into the PCP lifestyle. PCP is most likely to be taken with alcohol or marijuana, but chronic users come ultimately to prefer PCP alone.

The drug experiences of chronic PCPers vary greatly. Some have a long history of multiple drug abuse, while others have had little experience with other drugs.

The polydrug PCPer is likely to have been taking drugs for several years, either as recreation or self-medication for underlying problems (18–20). This individual often finds PCP the best of all possible drug worlds because it tends to relieve the user's anxiety and pain. Some even claim that it solves their problems with other drugs. We have seen several heroin addicts convert from methadone to PCP as a preferred method of abstinence from heroin, and a number of chronic alcoholics claim that PCP removes their desire for alcohol. Such substitutions, reminiscent of the use of heroin in the early 1900s to "cure" alcoholism, more often than not lead to further complications.

From our discussions with users and those who treat them, it appears that the new generation of PCPers is less experienced with drugs. Alcohol and marijuana appear to be the only consistent prerequisites to experimenting with PCP. Familiarity with the ritual of smoking marijuana certainly contributes to experimenting with PCP. The majority of PCP experimenters say they believe that any drug that can be smoked poses no great hazard.

Most chronic PCPers started using the drug in a social setting, and they continue to use the drug socially. Approximately 85 percent of the chronic PCPers we've studied were introduced to the drug by a group of friends. The family house is the most common site for such gatherings of two to five youths. PCP often becomes the common denominator or cement that keeps the group cohesive over time. While intoxicated on PCP, the group listens to music, talks, dances, and on occasion indulges in sexual activity. PCP is used as often during the daytime as the evening. PCPers are likely to stay at home rather than go out in public, in part because they fear coming into contact with the police.

A unique feature of the PCP lifestyle is the almost familylike atmosphere of the peer group. A truly sharing and caring relationship dominates the dynamics of the group. The loyalty among chronic PCPers is not found with other drug abusers, who have much more fragile relationships. It is our impression that a heroin addict who overdoses is much more likely to be victimized by his peers than is an unconscious PCPer. Members of the PCP group appear to look out for one another. Those who are depressed or on a bad trip are usually kept with the group until they recover. Group members generally have easy access to the drug through manufacturing or dealing, thus eliminating many of the interpersonal conflicts seen among heroin addicts.

As chronic PCPers increase their use of the drug, they become more isolated, moving toward a solitary pattern of intoxication. Eventually they disassociate from the group, and all interpersonal relationships break down. At this point serious problems emerge in their jobs, marriage or significant-other relationships, and self-concept.

## Profiling the PCPer

Our study of PCPers has led to several general findings.

☐ The majority of young people consider PCP the next step up from marijuana. It is estimated that 43 million Americans have tried marijuana, and it is assumed that as many as 11 percent of all high-school seniors use it daily (21). PCP represents an attractive new drug experience for what could be a tremendous number of Americans (12,13).

☐ First-time PCPers are usually introduced to the drug through friends in a small group. Using the drug alone may represent the threshold where true interpersonal problems begin, since the user's desire for intoxication must outweigh fear of the consequences of taking the drug alone (12,13).

☐ Chronic PCPers are no less intelligent than nonusers, but as evidenced by school performance and occupational goals, they are underachievers. Personal and social anomie are directly related to PCP abuse (17).

☐ The musical tastes of PCPers first tended to be hard rock and punk rock and now run to disco. Interestingly, PCP abuse rose suddenly in Great Britain just before the punk rock movement and may have supported the evolution of this musical form (22).

☐ Sensation seeking is a dominant force in the lives of chronic PCPers. The drug tends to remove inhibitions, unleashing risk taking that PCPers themselves find incredible after the fact. Risk taking likely contributes to using the drug in the first place. One study found that 86 percent of chronic PCPers believed the drug dangerous, yet they continued to use it (17). PCPers may take the drug just so they can boast about it later. Several PCPers have confided to us that they continued to use the drug after a life-threatening overdose as a way of defying death.

☐ If they survive the hazards of repeated intoxication, some chronic PCPers "mature out" of using the drug by their mid-twenties because they need lasting interpersonal and occupational involvement and psychological stability.

## PCP Abuse and Sexuality

Most abused drugs affect sexuality to some degree, and PCP is no exception. This effect arises in part because of the age of most PCPers. The teen-age years are filled with pronounced sexual changes, conflicting social signals, confusion, rebellion, and guilt. Sexually, PCP is a mixed blessing. The drug does allay anxieties about sexual development — changes in the body, maleness and femaleness, and high libido. Girls in particular find PCP a quick solution to their sexual confusion. They have more expectations about love, romance, and sex than boys and thus suffer more from interpersonal conflict, anxiety, and disappointment. However, despite its initial promise to the user, PCP finally interferes with sexuality.

As the new decade begins, the PCP analogs Ketamine and PCPY are becoming more popular because of their supposedly aphrodisiac effects on women only. This property of the drugs is not well documented or understood.

## Disinhibition

PCP helps remove inhibitions about sex. When asked to describe the effects of PCP on their sexual behavior, women said:

The first effect is a buzzing in my ears and slight pressure on my head — both pleasant sensations. From there it spreads throughout my whole body and the pleasantness increases. Then my thoughts loosen up. I get less inhibited and do things I ordinarily would not do or even think about.

I am not really the type of person who runs around showing off my body and yell and be loud. I would go dancing and get loaded, drive to places and not remember how I got there or what I did. I would sometimes come home without my shoes.

I enjoy masturbating more on PCP. I can get into more fantasy trips. Although I enjoy it, I still prefer a man.

PCP's disinhibitory effects may be the single most important effect on female sexual behavior. Many have become the victims of "chemical rape" or seduction while intoxicated by the drug. Because PCP causes disinhibition and increases suggestibility, many young people describe the drug as an aphrodisiac.

I've seduced a lot of women with PCP. For example, I met this girl in a park. We got real loaded and my intentions were to get her high and take advantage of her. We just started hugging and kissing and got right into it. She went right along with me.

We were out in front of someone's house leaning against a cyclone fence in broad daylight. I had the urge and since we were both loaded, she more than I, I unzipped her pants and we did it while a big crowd stood around watching.

## Sexual Functioning

In *Macbeth* Shakespeare says of alcohol's effect on sex, "It provokes the desire, but it takes away the performance." By and large this is true of all psychoactive drugs taken in sufficient quantity. PCP is no exception. It increases interest yet diminishes performance.

The young male attempting to overcome premature ejaculation may consider PCP the answer due to its anesthetic effects. However, since the properties of the drug are dose specific, the premature ejaculator may find PCP advantageous one time and totally unsatisfactory the next. Often the drug prevents erection, and repeated failures may well contribute to the onset of impotence, which commonly follows premature ejaculation.

For women, who tend to be more emotionally invested in their sexual relationships than men, PCP may chemically mediate emotional conflict. The total impact on female sexual behavior and functioning is really not clear, however.

Both men and women experience occasional subjective improvements in their orgasmic response. Whether their orgasm is indeed improved or whether their perception of orgasm is simply altered is unknown. Indeed, PCPers often report that they cannot have an orgasm while intoxicated. Some have engaged in intercourse for hours without climaxing. Some women who are highly orgasmic report themselves unable to climax while on PCP. Others reach an orgasm they think better than usual yet remain dissatisfied by their inability to feel general body contact because of PCP's partial anesthetic effect.

In one study of chronic PCPers, only 57 percent of the users reported satisfactory sex lives (17). It appears that PCP confers no lasting benefits on sexual functioning. This is hardly surprising. Sex is largely a function of the mind, and PCP is a mind–altering drug. PCP also causes interpersonal relationships to deteriorate, and this is bound to affect sexual functioning, since reciprocity and sensitivity to the partner's sexual needs are harmed by the drug.

In sum, PCP appears to be a barrier to a healthy sexual lifestyle. As one PCPer put it, "PCP replaces sex when you get heavy into using. On PCP you become completely self–centered around common pleasures."

# 34    PCP, Brain Damage, and Aggression

Both PCPers and others concerned with the angel dust problem often ask whether PCP causes long-term and lasting damage to the brain. The question is important. PCPers often say they hear their "brains frying," and some figure that if the damage has already been done, there is no reason for them to stop using the drug.

A study to assess the effects of PCP on cognitive and personality functioning compared a group of fourteen PCPers who averaged three years of regular exposure with a matched group of controls who reported never having used PCP (17). Both groups, averaging 20.9 years of age, were screened to rule out head injury, seizure disorder, psychiatric hospitalization, and psychotherapy. At the time of testing all subjects were oriented and not under the influence of PCP as determined by standard clinical tests. The study's findings are revealing.

☐   No statistically significant differences in general adult intelligence (IQ) appeared between PCPers and controls.

☐   Differences in group averages on short-term memory tests were also statistically insignificant.

☐   Significant differences appeared in projective test results (Rorschach). Briefly, PCPers had difficulty controlling their emotions and repressing disruptive thoughts from their subconscious. Consequently, they may have been unable to control emotional outbursts. PCPers were more likely to form conclusions with little or inaccurate information. Therefore, as PCPers attempted task-oriented activities, the potential that disruptive material would come into consciousness and throw them off balance was very high, particularly when they were under stress. When asked if they had difficulty with figures or directions after taking the drug, 86 percent of the PCPers indicated they did. Also, 86 percent claimed they had peculiar or strange experiences. These two results varied from the nonuser group by a twofold amount.

☐   Statistically significant differences were found in major personality characteristics affecting social interaction. The PCPers' results on the MMPI showed significantly more psychopathology. They could be described as irritable, hostile, suspicious, and emotionally inappropriate, with a tendency toward acting out.

There is no conclusive evidence of brain damage from chronic **35** exposure to PCP. Also, since both users and controls varied similarly, it appears that the drug does not affect a specific area of psychological functioning. The major conclusion of this study is that PCPers are unpredictable, a finding corroborated by the professional experience of human service providers with PCPers. In addition, the unpredictability of PCPers is compounded by their inability at times to correctly perceive and interpret the situation.

The aggressiveness associated with PCP use may in part be understood by looking at the drug's effects on the user's drives and inhibitions (23). Stimulants increase drives, and depressants, such as alcohol and barbiturates, remove inhibitions, both leading to aggression. On the other hand, depression or passive behavior results from increasing inhibitions with drugs like lithium or from reducing drives with a drug like heroin. The unique properties of PCP — increasing drives and releasing inhibitions — increase the likelihood of aggressive behavior.

In a recent study of sixteen chronic PCPers, violent acts associated with PCP and alcohol intoxication were more likely to result from PCP or the combination of the two drugs than alcohol alone. Three of the sixteen subjects performed self-destructive acts while on PCP. Ten subjects gave accounts of twenty violent acts toward others, whereas six PCPers were victims themselves of violent acts. One was raped, one was hit by an automobile, and four were beaten (24).

In another study of nine PCPers, four of the six who committed acts against others committed violent offenses (one robbery, one rape, and two assaults). Five of the nine PCPers had attempted suicide (25). These studies parallel our observations.

## What PCP Costs the User

It is our experience and opinion that no street drug in so little time has taken a greater toll in life and suffering than PCP. Unfortunately, given PCP's relative novelty on the drug scene, the data are few and far between, often unreliable, and generally too conservative. Still, the figures show something of the cost in physical and mental ill health and even death to PCPers.

A survey of a small number of hospitals in ten major United States cities in six-month periods in 1976 and 1978 showed a dramatic increase in emergency-room cases treated for PCP toxicity (26).

| Location | 1976 | 1978 |
|---|---|---|
| Boston | 7 | 24 |
| Buffalo | 2 | 24 |
| Chicago | 64 | 118 |
| Los Angeles | 111 | 502 |
| Miami | 4 | 110 |
| New York | 1 | 67 |
| Philadelphia | 24 | 65 |
| Phoenix | 2 | 37 |
| Seattle | 6 | 34 |
| Washington, D.C. | 37 | 124 |

In every hospital, PCP cases increased markedly — from a low of 300 percent to a high of 6600 percent. Remember, too, that these figures take in only the diagnosed PCP cases. As Chapter 1 mentioned, the problem is often missed. There were almost certainly more PCP emergency-room cases than these figures indicate.

Mental institutions have also seen a wave of PCP abusers. For example, a large psychiatric facility in urban southern California reported that of the 1000 patients admitted each month between December 1977 and December 1978 as many as half had problems arising from PCP abuse (14). Unlike most toxic psychoses, PCP cases required two weeks of aggressive inpatient treatment before any positive results were seen (15,16).

Misdiagnosis of PCP toxicity is a problem in the mental institution just as it is in the emergency room. Because of the remarkable clinical similarity of the two problems, schizophrenia is the most likely misdiagnosis for PCP psychosis. Thus it is likely that the threefold increase in admissions for schizophrenia reported by a community mental health center in Washington, D.C., was due not to an epidemic of mental disorder but to the spread of PCP abuse (16).

PCP also causes death, again to a far greater extent than we realize. Our survey of one coroner's office in each of twenty states **37** found that 75 percent routinely tested for PCP in all autopsies.

| Location | PCP Included in Standard Drug Screen | Analogs Included | PCP-Related Deaths |
|----------|----------|----------|----------|
| Alaska | Yes | No | No |
| Arizona | Yes | ? | No |
| California | Yes | No | Yes |
| Colorado | No | No | ? |
| District of Columbia | Yes | No | Yes |
| Florida | Yes | Limited | Yes |
| Hawaii | No | No | Yes |
| Indiana | Yes | No | Yes |
| Kansas | Yes | ? | No |
| Louisiana | No | No | Yes |
| Massachusetts | Yes | No | Yes |
| Missouri | Yes | Limited | No |
| Nebraska | Yes | Limited | No |
| New Jersey | Yes | No | Yes |
| New York | Yes | Limited | ? |
| North Carolina | No | No | No |
| Ohio | Yes | No | Yes |
| Tennessee | Yes | Limited | Yes |
| Texas | Yes | Limited | Yes |
| Virginia | Yes | Yes | Yes |

Unfortunately, methods of analysis vary, probably accounting for many missed PCP deaths. In addition, while PCP analogs have become more popular, screening for these drugs is limited — less than 10 percent — further undercutting the validity of PCP testing. Also, as medical examiners and coroners have become aware of the bizarre circumstances surrounding PCP deaths, many have gone back to their records and reevaluated cases, with laboratory verification finding that deaths originally attributed to unknown causes were in fact due to PCP.

To us the most alarming aspect of the PCP problem is the self-mutilation, suicide, and homicide related to chronic abuse of the drug. We have assisted in the litigation of over one hundred PCP-related homicides since 1976. The typical defendant was a polydrug abuser who had started with glue sniffing at the age of twelve or thirteen.

## What PCP Costs the Community

When PCPers kill or mutilate themselves or turn their violence against others, the community ultimately pays — the immediate families in terms of financial loss and emotional trauma, and the community in terms of direct and indirect costs. Today, with NIDA conservatively estimating that 7 million Americans have sampled PCP, those costs mount to staggering sums.

Several independent studies report that it takes from $10 to $100 a week to support a chronic PCPer, with $50 being the average (9,12, 17). About one-third of the PCPers get their money illegally, usually by stealing or dealing. Making and dealing PCP has grown into a vast underground industry, where millions of dollars change hands without any return to the community through taxes. To give an idea of just how large this economy is, raids and seizures in the first six months of 1979 netted 42 illegal laboratories, 315 arrests, and 3,769,000 dosage units of PCP (22).

The medical costs of PCP abuse, which are often borne by the community, can be terrific. Many PCPers end up in hospital emergency rooms, at an average cost of $45 per visit. Acute toxicity can require as much as six weeks of hospitalization, with the total bill not uncommonly hitting $40,000. Chronic PCPers average two hospital stays. The legal costs of PCP can be equally fearsome. Litigating one PCP-related homicide costs from several thousand dollars to $1 million. The cost continues if there is a conviction. In California, as one example, a year's stay in jail costs more than $24,000.

In addition, the community is also losing money indirectly. The manufacture and trade of PCP is illegal and underground, with not a dollar of the many millions that change hands ever going back to the community in the form of taxes.

PCP exacts other costs. The laboratories often cause fires and explosions (27). The drug also disrupts the economy by removing workers, such as human service providers injured by violent PCPers and pilots unable to fly because of surreptitious PCP intoxication.

Finally, there is the loss of human potential. Every chronic PCPer represents a possible productive and involved member of the community lost to drug abuse. For that cost there is no accurate accounting.

## The Missing Pieces of the PCP Puzzle

For a drug that causes as much tragedy as PCP does, strikingly little is known about it. We mentioned earlier, for example, how the site of PCP's activity in the brain remains a mystery. That is but one of the missing pieces of the PCP puzzle. There are others.

□ We know from laboratory studies that PCP passes from the mother to the fetus. Further research is needed on the effects of the phencyclidines on fetal development and infant health as well as fertility.

□ Knowing the effects of phencyclidines on the total psychology of PCPers would provide a much better understanding of the relationship of PCP toxicity to learning and personality development.

□ Preliminary studies by coauthor Burns at the National Institutes of Health indicate that PCP's metabolites — that is, the breakdown products of the drug in the body — may be psychoactive and related to aggressive behavior in humans. Further research is needed to clarify this relationship.

□ That PCP interacts with other drugs is known but not understood. Since the vast majority of chronic PCPers are multiple drug abusers, the importance of understanding the mechanism and implications of combinations of the phencyclidines and other drugs cannot be overstated.

□ The sensitivity and reliability of screening methods for PCP have improved significantly over the past ten years. Additional research is required to expand these methods to include the commonly abused analogs of PCP.

**40**

☐ A specific compound to reverse the effects of PCP — an antagonist — would be a major contribution.

☐ The effects of high doses of PCP and chronic intoxication need further investigation. Emphasis should be placed on the relationship between abnormal behavior and chronic PCP use.

☐ The mechanism of toxicity and the means by which the phencyclidines and their precursors are distributed and metabolized within the body are critical questions that must be answered in order to better understand the relationship between the phencyclidines and their effects.

☐ Interdisciplinary research efforts are required to identify and control the causes of PCP abuse.

What we do not know about PCP exceeds what we know, and it is likely to be years before we learn what we still need to find out.

## Summary

Psychoactive drugs alter the functioning of the brain by changing that organ's natural biochemistry. The effect of the drug depends on the site of its activity within the brain.

PCP is a unique drug, with effects that resemble those of uppers, downers, and outers. The diagnostic symptoms of PCP intoxication are nystagmus and elevated blood pressure. The precise site of PCP activity is unknown.

PCP varies in risk from occasional experimental use to chronic use. Behavioral toxicity is always a threat, though, particularly for those intoxicated surreptitiously or accidentally.

PCPers find the drug experience pleasurable and exciting. Religious and death experiences are common, as are sensations of floating and of omnipotence. Severe acute depression is the most serious and potentially dangerous effect. The motive force behind PCP use seems to be the desire to escape.

Most PCPers have used other drugs first, but often their only experience is with alcohol and marijuana. The drug is usually used socially, and the group stays at home. The peer group is supportive **41** and familylike. Long-term PCP use leads eventually to social isolation and solitary intoxication.

The typical PCPer considers the drug the next step up from marijuana, uses it socially, is no less intelligent than nonusers but is an underachiever, likes hard rock or disco, is given to sensation seeking, and may stop using the drug by the mid-twenties because of changing psychological needs.

PCP helps remove inhibitions against sex, but the drug may interfere with sexual functioning. Although some users report superior orgasms, climaxing under the drug's influence can be difficult. The drug also undercuts interpersonal relationships, decreasing sexual reciprocity.

PCP causes no proven brain damage. Psychologically, PCPers are distinguished only by their emotional unpredictability.

Users of PCP faced increased risk of mental and physical ill health and death. The toll from these causes is underestimated.

PCP costs the community in terms of lost income, welfare and public medical costs, crime spawned by the PCPer's need to support the drug habit, untaxed income in the illegal manufacture of PCP, and harm to human service providers and others.

Important information about PCP, from effects on the unborn fetus to interactions with other drugs, still needs to be discovered.

42  **PART II**

RECOGNIZING
AND
MANAGING
PCP ABUSE

**CHAPTER 3**

RECOGNIZING
THE PCPer

To recognize the PCPer, you must understand the forms the drug takes on the street, its relative strengths and effects, and the patterns of its abuse. This chapter sets out guidelines for recognizing the PCPer drawn from our research and experience in collaboration with several thousand human service providers. We start with general indicators of PCP abuse for all human service providers, then focus on specific clinical benchmarks for health professionals.

**43**

## The Forms and Methods of PCP Use

Knowing what PCP looks like and how it is used can help human service providers recognize PCPers (1–11).

### The Forms of PCP

In the early days of the PCP movement, the drug came in tablets or capsules. This form entailed a distinct risk, since the tablet or capsule had to be taken all at once but its exact dosage was unknown. Some were found — usually by coroners — to contain lethal doses of phencyclidine (7).

PCP material ranging from a powder to a solid is usually called crystal. High-quality PCP often appears in a rocklike form that, like common table salt, lets light through. Crystal PCP replaced capsules and tablets because the powder can be sprinkled on leaf materials — bay, oregano, mint, parsley, and tobacco, for example — and smoked, allowing better control of dosage. This method also expanded the PCP movement because people already used to smoking marijuana or tobacco found it easy to use PCP. PCP sprinkled on leaf material is commonly called angel dust, and the mint aroma sometimes attributed to the drug in fact comes from the mint leaves, not the PCP.

In the mid-1970s liquid PCP gained popularity because of its higher potency and greater ease of use. PCP dissolved in various liquids looks clear or yellow, but sometimes dealers color the liquid to change its appearance. Liquid PCP is sprayed, sprinkled, or soaked onto leaves that are dried for smoking in a pipe or joint. Some PCPers soak a string in liquid PCP and thread it through conventional cigarettes to reduce their chances of being caught in possession of the drug. Liquid PCP can also be injected.

## How PCP Is Packaged

PCP is typically packaged in foil, plastic bags, vials, and paper packets or bindles. Foil and plastic are used because of the mistaken belief that the drug loses potency if it dries out. Glass or plastic vials are used for both liquid and crystal PCP. The paper bindles vary from homemade packages folded from ordinary writing paper to commercially manufactured products that are prefolded and lined with plastic.

PCP is also marketed as a "pinwheel" joint, a tightly rolled cigarette much smaller than a marijuana joint. Commercial cigarettes dipped in liquid PCP provide another type of packaging. Because white cigarette paper is thin and easily discolored by the PCP, dark-papered cigarettes are preferred.

PCP has even been carried into restricted settings like jails in a variety of ingenious ways: by soaking envelopes, letters, facial tissues, toilet paper, toothbrushes, dental floss, or package wrapping with liquid PCP, by hiding it in the lining of clothing, by putting a small quantity of crystal PCP under the postage stamp of a letter.

## How PCP Is Taken

PCP can be taken in a great variety of ways. The method a particular user favors depends on the form of the drug, the user's previous drug experience, and the ease of preventing an overdose with that form of the drug.

*Smoking.* Smoking is the most common way to take PCP. Since the majority of PCPers smoke marijuana or tobacco, smoking is a familiar and comfortable experience, and it buttresses the notion that PCP cannot be too much different from marijuana. "I like the taste of mint leaves" is a common reason given for smoking PCP. Others like the control smoking gives them: "It's too hard to tell how strong it is when snorting or swallowing. I've overdosed that way."

**45**

*Snorting.* PCP can be snorted, or inhaled, like cocaine, and this method is popular among those experienced with that drug. The ritual of preparing crystal PCP for snorting is much the same as for cocaine. Individuals who dislike smoking also tend to snort: "I like the taste and the feeling, a little bit of a burn and flavor."

*Swallowing.* Only novices and risk-taking chronic PCPers swallow the drug. "I enjoy dropping a PCP tab or cap, since I never know when the 'high' will come on or how 'high' I'll get." A swallower has no way of knowing just how much of the drug has been ingested. Recently, for example, peanut butter chunks laced with lethal doses of PCP (over 1 gm) were sold in the New Orleans area. Oral ingestion is the principal cause of pharmacological deaths from PCP.

*Injection.* Our recent psychological study found that an increasing number of chronic PCPers are injecting the drug intravenously as their preferred method of use (2). Some of these PCPers have abused heroin or methamphetamine this way. "The rush is different, instant and more intense," claimed an ex-heroin addict and current PCPer. Some of the PCPers had not injected any other drug, however. A PCPer who had never before used a needle reported, "I like the rush. I don't get it from snorting or eating, plus you don't have the burning from snorting." Another PCPer said, "As expensive as it is, I don't want half of it going out my nose. I want to get my money's worth."

## Other Methods

Liquid PCP has been placed directly into the eyes with a common eyedropper. Individuals worried about the police use this method. One PCPer stated, "I've never had a cop check out my eyedrops."

**46**

PCP is also used rectally or vaginally, often for certain sexual practices. The drug's numbing effect throughout the body is conducive to anal intercourse and sado-masochistic sexual behavior. According to one user, "PCP, when used rectally, enables you to relax, to really get into it with little discomfort."

## Method and Dosage

The concentration of PCP varies with the form of the drug. The following figures give approximate values, which vary significantly from place to place (7,8).

| Methods/Forms Used | Estimated Amount of PCP |
|---|---|
| Smoking — joint | 5 mg |
| Snorting — powder | 5 mg |
| Swallowing — tablet/capsule | 5 mg |
| Injection — liquid | 10 mg |
| Eyedrops — liquid | Unknown |
| Rectally — liquid | Unknown |
| Vaginally — liquid | Unknown |

When PCP is smoked, only about 30 percent of the drug in the joint may actually enter the lungs. The remainder is lost to combustion. As a result, PCP smokers use more of the drug over the same length of time than those who favor other methods.

## Method and Effects

However PCP is taken, the drug's effects remain the same. What differs is the timing of the various events. Suppose that an individual takes two or three inhalations from a joint laced with about 5 mg of PCP (7, 8). The "high" begins in one to five minutes, and it **47** peaks, or hits a plateau, in fifteen to thirty minutes. The smoker stays "loaded" for four to six hours, and returns to predrug "normal" state in twenty-four to forty-eight hours. When injected, the effects begin in about the same time. When snorted or taken rectally or vaginally, there is a few minutes delay. Swallowed PCP does not produce effects for thirty to sixty minutes.

## Recognizing the PCPer

The first sign of PCP intoxication is bizarre or inappropriate behavior. The following incident is illustrative.

### Case # 1818.

On a jumbo airliner enroute to Honolulu on March 7, 1978, a passenger removed all of his clothes, stood up in the front of the cabin, and raised his arms. He claimed to have seen God and had to be natural. Refusing to get dressed or listen to the flight attendant, he was handcuffed and strapped in a row of seats. Two hours later he was allowed to sit up with his hands tied in front of him with pantyhose. He was quiet for the remainder of the trip. The flight attendant noticed nystagmus. It was reported later that he disrobed again in the baggage area.

Even behavior as bizarre as this is not a certain sign of PCP, since it could arise from intoxication by other drugs or psychosis, among other causes. But whenever PCP is suspected, other signs help substantiate the drug's presence.

Jerky movement of the eyes, or *nystagmus,* is the best single indicator of phencyclidine intoxication. When PCP intoxication is suspected, you should look first for jerky eye movements, or what is called nystagmus. You should test for nystagmus in horizontal and vertical directions.

To test for horizontal nystagmus, sit directly in front of the suspected PCPer. Point your finger straight up and hold it about 15 inches from the subject's nose and 1 or 2 inches above the eye level so that you can see the eyes. Ask the subject to hold his or her head still and follow your finger with his or her eyes. Then move your finger slowly 2 feet to the right or left in a straight line. The eyes of a subject on PCP will show nystagmus at the limit of their horizontal movement.

Even when you find horizontal nystagmus, you should also check for vertical nystagmus, which, in a conscious PCPer, rules out barbiturate toxicity. The procedure is the same, except that you move your finger up and down starting at the level of the nose.

The presence of both vertical as well as horizontal nystagmus is an almost certain sign of PCP intoxication. To verify the initial diagnosis, look for three other signs.

Incoordinated walking, or *gait ataxia,* can be determined by asking the person to walk a straight line by placing their feet heel to toe. The PCPer often has a *blank stare,* an expressionless face with unblinking eyes. This condition can be uncovered simply by observing the person's face briefly. Finally, the PCPer often has muscle rigidity, which makes itself evident to simple observation as a stiff appearance or unusual body posture.

When all these signs are present, you can assume phencyclidine intoxication. For additional confirmation, check the subject's blood pressure. PCP is the only abused drug that produces both nystagmus and elevated blood pressure. The amount of the drug needed to bring on these effects is enough to warrant referring the subject for observation or treatment.

## Questioning the PCPer

If the subject is cooperative, it pays to question him or her to determine as much as possible about the PCP taken as well as any other drugs that may have been used. These questions can prove helpful.

□     What did you take? **49**
□     How much did you take?
□     Do you have any of the drug left?
□     Can you describe what you took (i.e., color, smell, taste)?
□     How did you take it?
□     When did you take it?
□     Have you ever taken it before?
□     How do you feel?

## Toxicological Screening

Unfortunately, human service providers, even those aware of the PCP problem, can misdiagnose the condition. One study found that of sixty-one PCPers seen by human service providers, only eight, or 13 percent, were correctly diagnosed for PCP toxicity (4). The others' conditions were attributed to coma, trauma, meningitis, cardiovascular accident, various psychoses, organic brain syndrome, and alcohol intoxication. Misdiagnosis poses the threat of unnecessary and potentially dangerous medical procedures.

The following case illustrates why toxicological screening for PCP is important.

Case #1126.

A thirty-six-year-old white male was admitted to the psychiatric ward for suspected ingestion of approximately 100 mg of Valium. The patient's condition rapidly deteriorated. He lost consciousness and was transferred to the intensive care unit. The attending physician could not account for the patient's condition. He questioned the initial assumption that Valium alone was responsible for the symptoms. Ingestion of peraldehyde or antifreeze was then suspected. The patient died less than twenty-four hours after admission. Upon investigation ten months later, the forensic pathologist determined that the cardiopulmonary arrest was due to the effects of ingesting phencyclidine.

Any patient who is admitted to an emergency room for suspected drug ingestion or whose symptoms do not allow a definitive diagnosis should have a general toxicological screen that includes tests for the phencyclidines. A number of laboratory tests can be used to test for PCP: gas chromatography, thin-layer chromatography, gas chromatography/mass spectrometry (GC/MS), and radioimmunoassay (RIA) (12). The most specific and sensitive method is GC/MS. A recent clinical study found that thin-layer chromatography, the least sensitive method, detected PCP in only 15, or 8 percent, of 180 PCP-positive urine samples detected by GC/MS (13).

The clinical course of poisonings are generally related to blood levels of the drug involved. With PCP, most patients in coma have phencyclidine blood levels greater than 100 nanograms per milliliter (ng/ml). With blood levels in the range of 200 to 500 ng/ml, patients exhibit respiratory depression or seizure. Blood levels of 500 ng/ml to 5 micrograms per milliliter (mcg/ml) have been associated with death from the drug's pharmacological effects. Blood phencyclidine levels greater than 1 mcg/ml would be expected to result in death if the seizures were not controlled and respiratory support not given (5,6).

However, current analytical methods may not be sensitive enough to detect PCP levels as low as those found in the blood. Urine provides a better test for initial diagnosis since the drug concentrates there and levels are generally much higher than in the blood. Gastric fluid obtained by nasogastric suctioning or lavage can also be screened for the drug. Gastric fluid is likely to contain a higher level of PCP than the blood because of the chemical characteristics, namely the ion-trapping effect, of the acidic gastric fluid. Also, the more acidic the urine the greater the likelihood of detecting the presence of PCP.

Whenever a urine sample is taken for PCP testing, its acidity (pH) should be measured immediately because the pH of urine changes quickly at room temperature. The pH indicator slips used for routine urinalysis are adequate. The following approximate correlations between urine and serum of levels of PCP in various body fluids can be useful for medical and legal purposes (14). A psychotic patient with a PCP blood level of 20 ng/ml might erroneously be considered to have had the diagnosis of toxic PCP psychoses ruled out by a blood test run by a method with a lower sensitivity limit of 50 ng/ml, or a test run on a urine of pH8 (14).

| Body Fluid | pH | Ratio Fluid:Serum |
|------------|------|-------------------|
| Urine | 7.5–8.0 | 1:1 |
| Urine | 6.5–7.4 | 7:1 |
| Urine | 5.0–6.4 | 36:1 |
| Urine | <5.0 | 97:1 |
| Gastric | <2.5 | 42:1 |
| Gastric | >2.5 | 20:1 |

## Emergency Medical Diagnoses

A PCPer admitted to an emergency room may present a combination of symptoms that makes correct diagnosis difficult. Acute confusion or coma, however, usually implies drug intoxication. In the absence of focal neurological findings, the physician must rule out encephalitis, head injury, a postictal state, or metabolic cause. This already murky picture has been muddied further by the recent upsurge of accidental and surreptitious PCP poisonings of both adults and children. To diagnose properly, the physician should be familiar with the clinical pictures of the confused-excited state and prolonged coma induced by phencyclidine.

Ranged from mild to acute, the states of PCP intoxication include confusion, agitation, coma, and prolonged coma. The PCPer often vacillates between the confused and agitated states, and the patient coming out of coma often passes through the confused and agitated states (2,8–11).

## Confused and Agitated States

A PCPer who appears confused or agitated has taken approximately 5 mg of the drug. Peak blood levels would be predicted at 50 ng/ml. The characteristic signs of most PCPers in these states include:

☐ Horizontal and vertical nystagmus
☐ Gait ataxia
☐ Increased blood pressure

**52**

- ☐ Increased deep tendon reflexes
- ☐ Blank stare
- ☐ Lack of communication

This case exemplifies a typical instance of confusion and agitation from PCP intoxication.

## Case # 1107.

After smoking most of a PCP joint while seated in a bowling alley, the patient passed out and upon regaining consciousness was unable to speak. Police and paramedics were summoned. When seen in the emergency room, the nineteen-year-old male was unresponsive to questioning. His speech was slurred and he had difficulty expressing himself. Blood pressure was 162/90, pulse 69, respiration 24. The patient had disconjugate gaze and both horizontal and vertical nystagmus. Toxicology for PCP: urine, 0.5 mcg/ml. Fluctuating states of confusion and agitation prevailed for seven hours. Orientation and cooperation were maintained for two hours before discharge.

## Comatose State

On the average, taking 20 mg of phencyclidine induces coma. The predicted peak blood level would be 200 ng/ml, with recovery from the coma occurring when blood levels drop below 100 ng/ml. Phencyclidine toxicity in the unresponsive and immobile patient can generally be diagnosed by toxicological tests and physical examination. The characteristics of the comatose state are:

- ☐ Possibly open eyes
- ☐ Increased blood pressure
- ☐ Increased deep tendon reflexes
- ☐ Spontaneous nystagmus
- ☐ Muscle rigidity
- ☐ Diffuse theta and delta slowing on the EEG

A case involving the poisoning of a child with PCP provides a clinical picture of the comatose state.

**53**

## Case # 1175.

A twelve-month-old female infant was healthy until the evening of admission when she ate the butt of a cigarette, about 2 centimeters (cm) long, "laced with phencyclidine." She was active and alert for about an hour after ingesting the material. As she began to mumble and foam at the mouth, her mother noticed unusual eye movements and posturing. She was rushed to the hospital, where she was breathing intermittently. Intubated with difficulty, she had tonic upper extremities and flaccid lower extremities. After being placed on a respirator, she was transferred to a pediatric facility. On physical examination, she was comatose with spontaneous respiration, well nourished, well developed, and well hydrated. Blood pressure 100/50, pulse 120, respiration 30–35, temperature 98°F. Pupils equally reacted briskly at 4 millimeters (mm). Spontaneous nystagmus. She did not respond to pain. Vital signs and neurological state were monitored and samples drawn for toxicological screen. Within twelve hours spontaneous breathing resumed. Disorientation and irritability subsided after twenty-four hours. A phencyclidine urine level of 3.7 mcg/ml was evident at the time of admission.

The patient emerging from coma goes through the confused or agitated state before returning to normal.

## Prolonged Comatose State

The prolonged comatose state is uncommon, since the PCPer must take 70 to 200 mg or more of the drug to induce it. Blood concentrations in excess of 100 ng/ml persist for several hours to several days. The clinical signs of the prolonged comatose state are:

☐ Persistent increased blood pressure
☐ Extensor posturing
☐ Seizures

**54**   ☐   Hypoventilation or apnea
☐   Diffuse slowing and periodic slow-wave complexes on the EEG

The trauma that often accompanies PCP toxicity can complicate the diagnostic picture, as exemplified by this case.

## Case # 847.

An unconscious twenty-one-year-old male was brought from a community drug treatment program to the emergency room. He was comatose. There was a large hematoma over the right eye and the left eye was closed, but there were no other signs of trauma. Both pupils at 4 mm responded slowly to light; negative doll's eyes. The right ear had blood in the canal. Right focal seizures in arm and head were frequent, and there was one generalized seizure, yet the patient breathed on his own. Blood pressure was 154/94, pulse 92, respiration 20, temperature 99.6°F. The pattern of deep tendon reflexes was

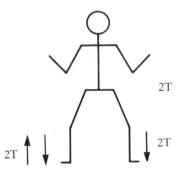

The attending physician diagnosed the situation as (1) subdural or epidermal hematoma, (2) PCP overdose, or (3) seizures, probably secondary to (1) or (2). The treatment plan called for an emergency cerebral angiograph, intubation, supportive IV fluids, lumbar puncture, and toxicology panel. Carotid arteriogram ruled out subdural hematoma. Lumbar puncture ruled out meningitis. Patient given Dilantin for seizures. Patient continued in coma for five days at which time pneumonia and phlebitis developed and were treated successfully. Patient regained consciousness and recovered uneventfully.

The patient's physical appearance suggested that his symptoms were due to head injury, but a subsequent history revealed that it was a mixed picture he had "also eaten some PCP." The black eyes were a diagnostic dilemma; they came from a fight two days before the PCP episode.

**55**

A prolonged and fluctuating state of confusion should be anticipated in a patient recovering from a massive overdose of phencyclidine.

## Differential Diagnoses

Other medical problems may accompany PCP toxicity. We have already seen how trauma can complicate the picture. In addition, since PCPers are often polydrug abusers, other abused drugs must be considered (2,5,9–11).

Probably the clinical characteristic that most distinguishes PCP intoxication from other forms of drug intoxication is vertical nystagmus, which appears even with low levels of PCP. A blank stare appearance and muscle rigidity are often associated with the nystagmus. Central nervous system stimulants and LSD can be ruled out in an excited or confused patient with nystagmus, and ataxia. If the pupils are not constricted, opiate intoxication can be ruled out.

Phenytoin and Wernicke's encephalopathy as well as PCP intoxication produce confusion, vertical nystagmus, and gait ataxia. There are differences, however. In phenytoin intoxication, but not in PCP intoxication, the upper extremities are pronouncedly incoordinated. Wernicke's syndrome also commonly involves lethargy and paralysis of the eye muscles. In addition, the patient often has a history of alcoholism and malnutrition.

In a comatose patient with nystagmus and muscle rigidity, phencyclidine should be suspected. If the patient is hypertensive and hyperflexic, whether respiratory depression is present or not, an overdose of sedative hypnotics can be ruled out. Cerebellar hemorrhage may mimic phencyclidine toxicity, but it lacks the diffuse theta activity and periodic slow-wave complexes that appear on the EEG with PCP intoxication.

Final diagnosis must be verified by toxicological screening and EEG.

## 56    Psychiatric Diagnoses

PCP offers a particularly perplexing problem for mental health personnel because behavior brought on by PCP intoxication often mimics mental illness. The psychosis arising from organic brain syndromes caused by PCP intoxication can last from several days to several months in both the first-time and chronic PCPer, and the condition is difficult to distinguish from schizophrenia. Since severe psychiatric disorders can arise even when there is no detectable level of PCP in the body, the patient's history may be crucial in differential diagnosis. Toxicological tests, however, should always be made upon admission (5,10,11,14).

The presenting symptoms of PCP psychosis and schizophrenia do differ subtly. This list compares the symptoms of each; + stands for sometimes, ++ for often, +++ for usually, and ++++ for always (15).

|  | Phencyclidine | Acute Schizophrenia |
|---|---|---|
| Autistic dreamy states | ++++ | ++ |
| Concrete thought | ++++ | ++ |
| Depersonalization | ++++ | +++ |
| Attention disorder | +++ | +++ |
| Clouding delirium | +++ | + |
| EEG changes | +++ | rare |
| Affect disorder | ++ | ++++ |
| Ambivalence | ++ | +++ |
| Catatonia | ++ | + |
| Loosened association | ++ | ++++ |
| Overinclusive thoughts | ++ | ++++ |
| Response to isolation | ++ | ++ |
| Delusional thinking | + | ++++ |
| Feelings of influence | + | ++++ |
| Visual hallucinations | + | rare |
| Withdrawal | + | +++ |
| Chlorpromazine response | +(?) | +++ |
| Intensified by amphetamine | +(?) | +++ |
| Cardiovascular and motor changes | marked | maybe |
| Auditory hallucinations | rare | + |

A recently intoxicated PCP patient may show nystagmus and the **57** other general diagnostic signs discussed above. Other mental signs can be used to help differentiate PCP intoxication from schizophrenia.

PCPers lack an organized symbolic process. In schizophrenics fragments of paranoia or religiosity are more disorganized. Importantly, the delusional states of PCPers are less systematized and disintegrate faster than those of schizophrenics. Paranoid ideation often lasts for long periods in PCPers. It is not uncommon for chronic PCPers to carry weapons to protect themselves from their imagined enemies.

PCP significantly alters the abusers' ability to determine time and to perceive depth. Memory is also disturbed, both short and long term. Cases we know of vary from one PCPer who could not remember where he had parked his car to another who could recall nothing of her early childhood.

PCPers' speech processes are often disrupted. Their speech pattern is fragmented, and they have difficulty articulating. One of the most obvious clues of PCP intoxication is stuttering, which leads to word substitutions.

PCPers grimace or clench their jaws. This indicates that they may unpredictably bite others or, less often, themselves.

PCPers' difficulty in perceiving and organizing physical experiences distorts the body image, leading PCPers to exaggerate the location, size, shape, and height of their bodies. Chronic PCPers report sensations of floating in and out of their bodies, an experience called astroprojection and brought on primarily by acute intoxication. Mind and body may dissociate, with PCPers viewing themselves from outside their bodies. The experience of a fourteen-year-old chronic PCPer is typical:

I was laying on my bed after smoking a PCP joint. I really thought I was dying. My mind left my body and went up into a corner of my bedroom. And I was watching myself as I stopped breathing. I kept telling myself from the corner of the room, "Come on, start breathing. You can do it, Come on. This will be the last time. I'll never take it again. Just wake up. Wake up." I was finally okay. It was a bad trip, yet I went back to smoking another joint the next day.

While under the influence, PCPers often see themselves as invulnerable, powerful, omnipotent, and physically and mentally superior.

Usually it is difficult if not impossible to communicate with intoxicated PCPers. Their delusional system is inconsistent and unpredictable, but familiarity with the delusional system of schizophrenics can make it easier to deal with the behavior and affective reactions of PCPers. Talkdown techniques used for "bad trips" during the LSD era do not work for PCP intoxication. Sometimes, in fact, they agitate the PCPer and may put the attending professional in danger.

Chronic PCPers are prone to acute depression, poor social adjustment, and psychological disorders that often precede their use of the drug. Suicidal risks are not uncommon. A lack of self-esteem is a major characteristic of this group of chronic drug abusers.

## Summary

Currently PCP is sold mostly as liquid or crystal. The drug is packaged in a variety of characteristic and sometimes concealing ways. It is taken by smoking, snorting, swallowing, injecting, dropping into the eye, or inserting into vagina or rectum. Method affects dosage and the timing of the drug's effects.

The PCPer can be recognized by bizarre behavior, horizontal and vertical nystagmus, gait ataxia, blank stare, and muscle rigidity.

A conscious and cooperative PCPer should be questioned to elicit information helpful in treatment.

Toxicological screening helps prevent misdiagnosis of PCP intoxication. The most sensitive method is gas chromatography/mass spectrometry. PCP can be detected in the blood, but higher and more easily detectable levels occur in the urine and gastric fluid.

Emergency medical diagnosis rests on recognizing the clinical picture of the various states of PCP toxicity. These include the confused-agitated state, coma, and prolonged coma.

Differential diagnosis of the PCPer can be important. Often the clinical picture is complicated by polydrug abuse and intoxication by other drugs besides PCP. Phenytoin intoxication, Wernicke's syndrome, and cerebellar hemorrhage may also mimic aspects of **59** PCP intoxication.

The mental health worker must distinguish PCP psychosis from schizophrenia. Mental symptoms, time and depth perception, speech, and self-perception differ in the two conditions. Communication with intoxicated PCPers is often impossible and sometimes dangerous.

# CHAPTER 4

# MANAGING
# THE
# PCPer

PCP is a unique drug with unique effects and hazards, and it poses **61** an equally unique challenge for human service providers. Tried and true ways of managing drug abusers and others needing first aid are simply ineffective for handling PCPers; they may actually threaten the lives of PCPer, care providers, and bystanders.

## Case # 2220.

Paramedics received a call for transport to a hospital. They found a young man unconscious from ingesting a large amount of PCP. The paramedics strapped the patient in a face-up position. Enroute to the hospital, the patient aspirated and died from suffocation.

This death by aspiration could have been prevented by placing the patient on his side or stomach. This case illustrates how human service providers must adapt to the new challenges presented by PCP. Indeed, mismanagement of PCPers has already prompted several malpractice lawsuits.

This chapter prepares human service providers for managing PCPers, provides guidelines for a variety of settings — law enforcement, emergency room, community drug treatment, mental health — and lists ways of reducing PCP hazards in high-risk settings.

Many of the cases given here may seem extreme, as if we have purposely selected the most lurid "war stories" to lend this chapter all the sensationalism it will bear. In fact, these cases have been chosen because they illustrate the areas of major concern. More important, they show strikingly that when PCP is mismanaged, such dire results are more the rule than the exception.

## General Guidelines for Managing PCPers

A number of basic rules and procedures apply to managing PCPers in all settings.

**62**    Use Extreme Caution

Always assume that PCPers are unpredictable because of the fluctuating effects of the drug. They have little or no awareness of the consequences of their behavior for themselves or others. Therefore, do not try to manage PCPers by yourself. Keep a close watch on PCPers from a safe distance. Expect periods of cooperation alternating with periods of aggressiveness. Give PCPers no other drugs. Clear the area of bystanders and of objects that could pose hazards. If you suspect a PCP laboratory, call the police or fire department. Since accidental intoxication is likely, handle nothing suspected of being PCP.

## Remove All Hazards

If you are in doubt about a situation, assume the worst — that PCP is involved. Next, identify anything and everything in the setting that could harm yourself, the PCPer, or bystanders. Analyze the surroundings by projecting yourself into the environment as an unpredictable PCPer.

The most obvious hazards are objects that PCPers can use to harm themselves or others. Cars are a good example.

## Case # 101.

After smoking one PCP joint and drinking one can of beer, a sixteen-year-old male drove into the rear of a dump truck parked on the side of a city street. He received minor injuries while his younger brother, sitting in the passenger seat, died at the scene. The remaining female passenger, fourteen years of age, was hurled from the back seat into the windshield, severely mutilating her face.

PCP-related accidents of this sort have increased as more and more youths abuse PCP.

Enclosed areas, where PCPers feel trapped or cornered, can **63** create danger for those attempting to help.

Case # 624.

A security guard discovered a twenty-three-year-old male inside the secured fenced parking lot of a baking company. The guard approached and asked the intruder what he was doing. "I am stronger than God," he replied. The guard noted that he was spaced out. The intruder then attempted to reach for the guard's revolver. The guard retreated and fired several rounds into the air as a warning. The intruder kept laughing and lunged at the guard, who in turn fired once into his chest. Continuing the attack, the guard fired again, fatally wounding the intruder.

If the guard had realized that he was dealing with PCP intoxication, he should have backed off and called for police assistance. Firing his weapon as a warning only further stimulated the PCPer, who may not have acknowledged how grave the situation was. PCPers often misinterpret what they perceive, and in the enclosed area the PCPer may have seen the guard as a threatening force whether he had a gun or not.

High places are hazardous for PCPers, who may not appreciate the ultimate — and fatal — consequences of a fall.

Case # 1556.

A male, twenty-six years of age, smoked five to six PCP joints at a friend's apartment. He had been smoking earlier that day and was a regular user. Without warning, he jumped out the second story window, landing on a fence before striking the ground. He then removed all his clothing and climbed the stairs of the apartment building onto a balcony. He then dove off the balcony onto the concrete below and died instantly. He had been taken to a local hospital by the police for irrational behavior and released earlier that same day.

Assume that all PCPers in areas of imminent danger behave irrationally. In such circumstances, an all-out effort should be made to restrain the PCPer.

Case # 131.

A twenty-seven-year-old woman, known to have used PCP regularly for four years, smoked one-half of a joint while putting on her swimsuit. She then dove into the backyard pool as her fiance was suiting up. She was found minutes later at the bottom of the pool and pronounced dead at the scene.

In the water PCPers may not be able to tell up from down, nor may they know where their arms and legs are in relation to their bodies. Therefore, it is important to warn young people to stay out of the water while they are on PCP (1,2).

Do not enter the water alone to help a PCPer in distress. Use alternate lifesaving techniques. If all else fails, tie a rope around the PCPer's waist, tie the other end to a fixed object, and pull the PCPer in.

Almost any body of water holds a danger to the PCPer. Users falling unconscious from PCP overdoses have drowned in only two or three inches of water.

Case #135.

A girl, seventeen years of age, was arrested for driving under the influence and resisting an officer. During the booking process she was left unattended in a shower. Later she was found dead with her body over the drain.

Had the arresting officers known the girl to be a PCPer, they would have obtained a medical clearance before booking and they would have seen that she should not have been left alone in the shower.

PCPers offer the greatest threat to others in crowds or large gatherings.

**65**

## Case # 1954.

During an annual celebration in Texas, a sixty-three-year-old man parked his camper along the parade route. As the participants passed, he began firing his rifle, killing three people and wounding fifty-five others. He was subsequently shot by police and found upon autopsy to have PCP in his system.

Assume that anyone whose behavior is bizarre and who has a weapon is a PCPer. Bystanders may be at risk because of PCPers' unpredictability and penchant for violence. It might seem best to evacuate all bystanders from the vicinity, but the sight of people running from the scene may stimulate PCPers. Therefore, it could be safer for bystanders to seek the nearest cover than to run. Do not attempt to intervene; call for police help.

Treatment and detention facilities are additional sources of danger to PCPers and others. A standard emergency room scenario begins when police arrive with a PCP-intoxicated youth in handcuffs. The patient may initially appear lucid and cooperative, and the physician, disliking the idea of treating a prisoner instead of a patient, demands removal of the handcuffs. The police warn the physician that the youth may be extremely hostile, but the doctor insists and they remove the cuffs. Then as the police are about to leave the hospital, the physician calls for them to stop the patient from dismantling the emergency room.

A life-threatening incident occurred in a medical holding cell.

## Case # 1701.

A young man brought in for acting bizarre was awaiting the jail physician. Upon hearing a strange gurgling sound, the nurse supervisor returned to find the man in the cell hanging upside down. He had tied his ankle to the cell bars.

With PCPers back-up support and constant monitoring must be maintained. Remember that PCPers may become depressed and suicidal at any time. Precautions should be taken against self-destruction.

## Administer Required First Aid

PCPers often come to the attention of human care providers while they are in need of emergency life-support care. If the victim appears unconscious, check to see whether he or she is breathing. If breathing has stopped, administer oral resuscitation. Be careful to avoid being bitten or poked in the eyes by a PCPer regaining consciousness.

You should also check for a pulse by gently placing the index and middle fingers over the carotid artery in the neck or the femoral artery in the groin. Do not use your thumb since the pulse you feel may be your own. If you find no pulse, begin cardiopulmonary resuscitation (CPR).

Look for signs of head, neck, back, or internal injuries. These often result from the behavioral toxicity of PCP, yet PCPers usually do not report them because the drug's anesthetic properties keep them from feeling any pain.

Unconscious victims should be placed on their sides so that vomit cannot enter the lungs. Transport PCPers in restraints on their side or face down.

## Reduce All Stimulation

PCPers react to stimulation, and the more they are stimulated, the more adversely they may react. Such reaction is most likely when the user is noncommunicative. Disorientation signals this state in the PCPer. You should back off until help arrives, and do nothing except to keep visual, auditory, and tactile stimulation to a minimum.

# Know Your Local Resources                                    **67**

Become familiar with the places where PCPers can get emergency medical treatment. Anyone under the influence of PCP should be cleared by a qualified physician, but some hospitals refuse to accept PCP patients. Find out which hospitals in your area will take them. You should also determine which local detoxification and habilitation program PCPers should be referred to after release by medical personnel.

## Law Enforcement Officers and the PCPer

The first wave of PCP abuse in the early 1970s caught law enforcement officers off guard. Early confrontations between peace officers and agitated PCPers indicated that traditional ways of controlling unruly suspects did not work and could prove very dangerous. This case history comes from the records of the California Highway Patrol.

## Case # 21.

On May 6, 1972, at approximately 1720 hours, . . . a nineteen-year-old was traveling on Lake Road near Turlock. The vehicle became disabled and [subject], along with two companions, began walking west. [The subject] apparently went berserk and threatened his companions. [He] attempted to strike the men with a tree limb; they became frightened and ran.

Approximately ten minutes later [a] traffic officer . . . came upon [the] subject walking in the center of the roadway. [The] officer . . . stopped the patrol car 20 to 25 feet to the rear of the subject to determine if he was in need of assistance.

Before the officer could exit, [the] subject . . . saw the patrol vehicle, ran to the right side, opened the front door, entered, and attempted to tear the shotgun from the Lektro-lok mounting. [The] officer . . . saw that the subject was grunting and groaning. The officer pushed [the subject] out the door. [The] officer . . . radioed, "11-99, I have a subject on a bad trip."

[The subject] ran around to the left side of the patrol car as [the] officer was completing his radio broadcast. [The subject] was ordered to the left of the road. [He] then attempted to forcibly enter the patrol vehicle through the driver's door.

The officer . . . pushed the subject away several times. [The subject] . . . started to walk away, enabling [the] officer . . . to obtain his baton. . . .

Again the subject attempted to enter the patrol car, forcing his way past the officer and trying to start the car. [The] officer . . . had previously removed the keys. Again [the subject] was pushed from the patrol car. [The] officer . . . was unable to restrain or control the subject. [The officer] radioed, "11-99, hurry up." [The subject] circled around the vehicle and assaulted the officer.

Three fishermen happened by the scene. They stopped to possibly render assistance. [The] officer . . . advised the fishermen of his problem and asked them to help him. [The] subject . . . had been calling out the name "Ray." [The] officer . . . , attempting to keep [the subject] away, told him to "go find Ray." [He] would not leave.

[The subject] continued his assault, causing the officer to use his baton. [The] officer . . . struck the subject across the hands and wrists several times. This did not affect [the subject]. The officer struck [him] solidly in the chest area with the end of the baton, again with no effect. [The subject] continued the assault; he was struck in the sides, [the] officer . . . swinging the baton in a full arc, using both hands with no effect. [The] officer . . . then struck the subject on the head across the temple area with no deterring effect.

[The subject] reached out and grabbed the baton with both hands. While the two men stood face to face grappling with the baton, [the subject] was lifting the officer off the ground and swinging him in an arc. Both individuals fell into a grassy ditch alongside the highway. The subject landed on top of the officer. [The officer] . . . called to the fishermen for help, and as they moved forward, the subject stood up. [The] officer . . . was then able to regain his footing; again he radioed an 11-99.

[The] subject . . . again attacked, and was successful in wrestling the baton away from the officer. Now swinging the baton, [the subject] advanced. [The] officer . . . was struck numerous times as he backed away. [The subject] began swinging at the officer's head. [The officer] . . . realized that if he was struck in the head and dazed or rendered unconscious, [the subject] would have access to his service revolver. The officer feared for the lives of the three fishermen as well as his own.

[The] officer . . . drew his service revolver, pointed it at the ground, and ordered the subject to throw down the baton. [He] . . . repeated the order while backing away as [the subject] continued the assault. [The] officer . . . fired two rounds at the subject's legs, hoping to disable him. One round struck [the subject] in the leg. [He] continued to aggressively swing the baton at the officer's head. A fourth shot [fired by the officer] struck [the subject] in the chest. [He] then went down to a sitting position. [The] officer . . . was carrying issue .38 caliber ammunition in a .357 magnum revolver.

An ambulance was requested. As the officer tried to control the bleeding, [the subject] attempted to continue his attack. [He] tore the bloody compress from his body and threw it at the officer, striking him in the chest.

An ambulance arrived and the subject was pronounced dead upon arrival at the hospital.

Upon autopsy, [the] body was found to contain PCP.

It is always easy to point out mistakes after the fact and say what should have been done instead. In this case, the officer had no idea what he was dealing with, and his usual ways of handling aggressive suspects brought injury to himself and death to the PCPer. This case and others like it have provided the fund of experience from which the current guidelines for handling PCPers by peace officers are drawn.

Two general points should be kept in mind. First, peace officers must remember that their own safety is essential to the safety of the public and the PCPer. If others are to be safe, the peace officers must remain in control of the situation. Losing control means that the PCPers may gain access to an officer's weapon, an outcome that usually ends in the use of deadly force.

Such tragedies stem primarily from the use of methods of control that work because they are painful. And that brings up the second point: because of PCP's anesthetic effects, pain-inflicting controls do not work. For example, the arm bar hold has at times brought death to either the officer, who loses control and becomes the PCPer's target, or the PCPer, who may suffer a broken neck. The carotid hold may work, but only if muscle rigidity has not affected the PCPer's neck. If it has, the hold is useless, and the officer who tries it may be hurt or killed. In fact, the carotid hold is more likely to fail than to work.

Various alternatives for controlling PCPers have been proposed, including nets and immobilizing agents. Here again, nothing is certain. Mace, for example, only stimulates PCPers, making a bad situation worse. Given the present state of knowledge and technology, we recommend these guidelines.

☐ When you suspect an agitated PCPers, call for help immediately Before any attempt is made to control the subject, there should be no fewer than five officers on the scene.

☐ Whenever possible, wait the situation out. PCPers behave unpredictably, and the aggressive PCPer may spontaneously become communicative and cooperative, ruling out the need for heroic intervention. Waiting it out is always a good strategy. It ensures that the PCPer has no access to an officer's weapon, thus preserving the safety of bystanders and officers alike. Besides, waiting is really the only alternative to deadly force.

☐ If you must gain control of an agitated PCPer, use the accumulative body-weight procedure. One officer sits on each limb while the remaining officer of the five prepares the subject for transport.

☐ If possible, transport the PCPer in an ambulance so that the subject can be held in the prone position with five-point restraints. If there is no ambulance, first handcuff the PCPer behind the back, then restrain the legs with a five-foot piece of one-inch nylon webbing with a slip loop at one end and a series of knots tied six inches apart at the other. Once the arms and legs are secured, place the PCPer headfirst on the back seat of the patrol car. To secure the webbing, place the knotted section over the top of the car door and close the door. When you reach the medical facility, remove the PCPer from the car by grasping the nylon webbing, then place the subject on a hospital gurney with five-point restraints.

A caution: do not underestimate the strength of a PCPer. Several violent PCPers have actually broken handcuffs that were not defective. Testing showed that breaking the cuffs by pulling them straight apart required a force of 1800 pounds per square inch and that at a 90° angle the cuffs had a tensile strength of 450 pounds per square inch. These are terrific forces, and PCPers who have broken handcuffs usually have also fractured their wrists or forearms. PCPers have even been known to pull the doors off patrol cars. To our knowledge, such behavior has never arisen from intoxication with drugs other than PCP.

☐ Suspected PCPers in the confused state should be handcuffed only and taken to a medical facility to be examined before they are detained. Treat comatose PCPers as medical emergencies requiring emergency life-support.

☐ Although all suspected PCPers should be cleared by a physician before booking and detention, they should still be routinely monitored. Suicidal behavior and self-mutilation in detention are not uncommon.

On the surface these procedures may seem to require an undue commitment of resources. But trying to handle PCPers with less commitment is a case of being penny wise and pound foolish. Cutting corners could cause the death of a PCPer, an officer, or a bystander, and the cost of that one lost life far exceeds the price tag of handling PCP situations with the care they deserve.

## Seizing and Taking Down the PCP Laboratory

Seizing and taking down a PCP laboratory is a hazardous undertaking. Certain of the chemicals they contain are highly explosive and toxic. The more dangerous chemicals and their effects are:

| Chemical Name | Appearance | Detection/Effects |
| --- | --- | --- |
| Piperidine | yellow liquid | Strong ammonia smell, soapy feel, obnoxious fumes. |
| Cyclohexanone | light yellow liquid | Peppermint and acetone odor. Irritation to eyes, skin, and mucous membranes; mild intoxication. |
| Sodium or potassium cyanide | chunky white crystalline substance | A bitter almond-scented lethal hydrogen cyanide gas may be generated when combined with hydrochloric acid. |
| Hydrochloric acid | clear liquid | Chlorinelike odor. Inhalation cough, choking, inflammation and ulceration of respiratory tract may occur. |

| Chemical Name | Appearance | Detection/Effects |
| --- | --- | --- |
| Ethyl ether | clear liquid | Mildly irritating to skin, mucous membranes. Inhalation of high concentrations causes narcosis, unconsciousness, possibly death. |
| Petroleum ether | clear liquid | Odor similar to white gasoline. Inhalation of high concentration causes headache, drowsiness, coma. |
| Magnesium turnings | silver metal | Inhalation of the dust irritating; metal fume fever; burns with a bright white flame. |

Thirty percent of the phencyclidine laboratories discovered make their presence known by exploding and burning, usually when a spark or flame ignites trapped hydrocarbons. The fire itself is a danger, plus some of the chemicals give off very toxic fumes when they burn. Magnesium turnings can explode when they come into contact with water. The most lethal gas, and one that commonly kills illicit PCP manufacturers, is hydrogen cyanide, which is produced when cyanide mixes with hydrochloric acid.

Before a PCP laboratory is seized and taken down, all personnel involved, including firefighters and criminalists, should be briefed. Follow these safety rules.

☐ Secure and evacuate the surrounding area.
☐ Have paramedics stand by.
☐ Have firefighters stand by. After the suspects are secure, firefighters should render the premises safe.
☐ Turn off gas and electricity at a source outside the premises.

☐     Use a gas probe to determine the fire potential inside the laboratory.     **73**

☐     Because of the fire hazard, allow no photography with flash units.

☐     Everyone entering the laboratory should wear self-contained breathing apparatus and helmet.

☐     A trained criminalist should always accompany investigators.

☐     The criminalist should shut down the operation and identify dangerous chemicals.

☐     The laboratory should be well ventilated by opening doors and windows. Mechanical ventilation equipment should only be used external to the location.

☐     The power should not be turned on again until the premises are well ventilated.

☐     No smoking.

☐     Thoroughly wash hands and change clothes upon leaving the site.

## Emergency Medical Treatment

In Chapter 3 we discussed how to recognize PCP intoxication. Once the condition has been diagnosed, emergency room personnel should be concerned primarily with life support, with protecting PCPers and others from behavioral toxicity, and with making the appropriate referral at discharge. Guidelines for achieving these goals reflect a combination of current research and clinical experience. There is no absolutely clear rationale of management nor conclusive validation. In their absence, we have developed procedures that are conservative and that minimize risks to patients.

These procedures are specific to the presenting clinical picture. You should always be prepared to alter the management plan as the clinical situation changes. Besides treating patients for PCP intoxication, you should also treat any other medical problems. Since PCP patients are unpredictable, you must be very cautious in implementing all procedures, avoiding instrumentation whenever possible. Ultimately, you have to rely on your training and clinical experience.

**74**     Treating PCP Intoxication

Since the treatment of PCP intoxication is essentially symptomatic, we will follow the major diagnostic categories of confused state, agitated state, comatose state, and prolonged comatose state.

*Confused state.*     Confused PCP patients should be placed in a darkened quiet room and constantly observed. Vital signs may be monitored, but all sensory stimulation should be kept to a minimum. Give confused PCPers a blanket. They often use it to establish a point of reference and to create a sense of boundary. A blanket helps calm PCPers in settings where they cannot be isolated.

The importance of constant observation cannot be overemphasized. The patient's state may vary, and one who initially appears stable can deteriorate seriously.

**Management of Confused State**

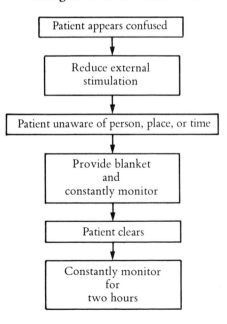

Case #1616.                                                    **75**

A twenty-eight-year-old white male was admitted for observation of bizarre behavior. After he was placed in a quiet room, he vacillated between cooperation and inappropriate, destructive behavior. About two hours later, a nurse found him hanging by a bedsheet.

All confused PCP patients should be monitored until they are alert, aware of person, place, and time, and behaving normally. However, patients released as soon as they are oriented often return because of subsequent episodes of abnormal behavior. Therefore, observe patients for two additional hours to rule out the recurrence of changed mental status.

Clinical studies have not shown that haloperidol and the phenothiazines shorten the recovery phase or antagonize the behavioral effects of the phencyclidines. The phenothiazines sometimes produce prolonged hypotension in confused PCP patients with hypertension, tachycardia, ataxia, and nystagmus (1). The phenothiazines may also lower the seizure threshold, adding further risk to PCP intoxication.

The confused patient who lapses into coma should be admitted to the hospital for medical observation. This change may signal the onset of life-threatening problems associated with progressive PCP toxicity.

*Agitated state.* Agitated PCPers often pose a serious threat to themselves and to others. Be prepared for aggressive or violent outbursts in all states of PCP intoxication, and particularly in agitated patients. Whenever the patient has a history of violence or is brought in by police, be ready to use restraints.

Three progressive stages of managing agitated PCPers are recommended. First, put the patient in a quiet room, preferably with a cushioned floor, and monitor (3). If the agitation lasts more than fifteen minutes, go to the next stage.

The second stage entails medicating the patient with 10 to 20 mg of diazepam orally (4). Clinical experience has shown that diazepam is effective in controlling behavior and that it does not produce complications. Repeated oral doses of 10 to 20 mg of diazepam may

## Management of Agitated State

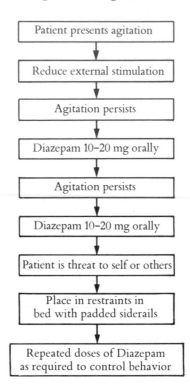

be necessary to control motor restlessness and agitation. If diazepam cannot be given orally, parenteral administration may be required (5–7).

The third management stage applies to patients so violent that they are a threat to themselves or others. Five-point restraints should be applied, and protective precautions, such as pads on the bedrails, should be taken. Should the patient remain agitated for another fifteen minutes, medication may be needed. Do not secure the restraints too tightly, since restraint of PCPers with increased muscle tone and activity has caused myoglobinuria with secondary kidney failure (1). Allow about six inches of movement under restraints, or place a mattress above the padded bed to allow mobility but keep the patient confined.

*Comatose state.*    Patients comatose from ingesting large doses of **77**
PCP often represent a medical emergency. Since large quantities of
unabsorbed PCP have been removed from the stomachs of victims
dead from overdose, the first procedure for comatose PCPers who
have ingested the drug orally is gastric aspiration and lavage. En-
dotracheal intubation is risky since it may precipitate laryngospasm. More responsive patients usually reject the procedure or
fight it by biting off the tube (3).

Muscle rigidity and myoclonic jerking may precede seizure activity. Intravenous diazepam in 2 to 5 mg increments effectively
controls the onset of phencyclidine-induced seizures. Manage seizure episodes separately with this treatment plan.

Respiratory status, urine color and output, temperature, and
blood pressure require routine monitoring (4). Red urine signals
myoglobinuria. Diazoxide has treated hypertensive crises effectively (8).

**Management of Comatose State**

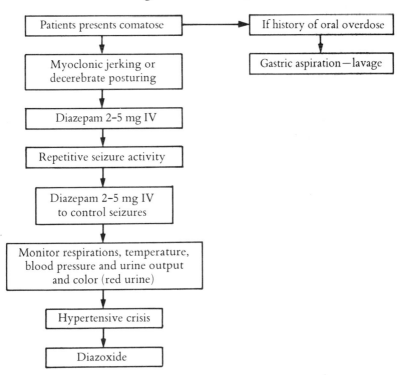

All phencyclidine patients in coma for more than two hours should be observed for a minimum of twenty-four hours (6,7).

*Prolonged comatose state.*　Massive oral overdoses of PCP usually result in a prolonged coma, which may last for more than two weeks. When patients regain consciousness, they may remain in the confused state. They are also subject to the same problems as comatose patients.

The prolonged comatose patients should be managed as comatose patients are. Specific procedures include ventilatory assistance for hypoventilation or apnea and positioning and intermittent suctioning to reduce respiratory distress secondary to secretions in the posterior pharynx (3,4).

A sustained increase in blood pressure can produce hypertensive encephalopathy (6,7).

## Ion Trapping – Acidification Treatment

There is no medication to alleviate the effects of the phencyclidines at present. In addition to symptomatic treatment, urinary and systematic acidification have been tried with acute PCP intoxication.

The rationale for urinary acidification rests on the fact that PCP is a weak base subject to pH-dependent urinary excretion. Since phencyclidine in the nonionized form is highly soluble in lipids, it easily passes through membranes, but when it is ionized, it loses solubility and passes through less easily. Acidic urine increases ionization, preventing the reabsorption of PCP back across the kidney membrane into the blood. As a result, more PCP than normal is excreted in the urine.

Systemic acidification also results in clinical improvement and maximal increases in urinary excretion of PCP, probably because this approach brings PCP out of the brain and other tissues into the blood, where it is eliminated through the kidneys. How effective acidification is in shortening coma and bringing the drug into the blood from the central nervous system has yet to be determined. We also do not know whether it is important that the procedure be begun at a particular time or whether aggressive acidification makes any difference (7).

## Discharge and Referral

All patients whose PCP intoxication has been confirmed should be warned that they may experience residual depression. "Post-phencyclidine depression" as late as forty-eight hours after patients are oriented to person, place, and time is not uncommon. Family and friends need to be informed about depression, irritability, feelings of isolation, and nervousness. At discharge, PCP patients should be referred to an appropriate drug or mental health program. The referral is likely to work best when drug or mental health personnel are involved in the predischarge process.

It is important that no PCP patient be discharged too soon. Mistakes can be tragic.

### Case #325.

A fifteen-year-old boy, reported to be a "troublemaker and out of hand," had been seen earlier in the month by a psychiatrist for depression and had talked about "getting it all over." The previous day he had been seen by an emergency room physician, who immediately released him. He was later found hanging by an electrical cord from a beam in his garage. PCP was the only drug found upon autopsy.

This case shows the importance of getting detailed information about drug patients before they are discharged. In this case, a thorough clinical evaluation, including drug history, may have alerted the attending physician to the patient's use of PCP and the need for referring the boy to mental health specialists. The boy's obvious depression should have received more professional attention, since PCPers become severely depressed and are likely to act on suicidal impulses.

PCPers can also hurt others, including their own children.

### Case #1501.

Neighbors heard a baby crying continuously for several minutes in an apartment and went to investigate. They discovered the twenty-three-year-old mother lying in a fetal position next to her infant son. She had taken a hammer and smashed each of her child's toes. Because of the extensive damage, nine of the toes were later amputated. This mother was booked and placed in a hospital jail ward. Upon regaining orientation, she had no recollection of the episode. Police found 5 ounces of a PCP analog in her living room.

This case underscores the importance of determining the living situation of PCPers before discharge. Whenever children are involved, be extremely cautious about returning them to the custody of a parent who uses or manufactures PCP. Spouses and neighbors merit the same concern.

Case #133.

The morning after smoking marijuana and PCP, a husband called for his wife to join him in their backyard. When she arrived, he proceeded to shoot her over twenty times with his semi-automatic rifle. As she lay dying, he turned the gun on his son, who managed to escape. A young boy riding by on his bicycle became the next victim. He was shot six times but lived. As the police drove up, a shootout resulted. Although hit in the exchange of gunfire, the man continued to advance toward officers until he finally dropped from the loss of blood. While the officers gave him first aid, he continued to resist. Upon recovering from his injuries, he had no recall of what had happened.

Both industry and military settings provide endless sources of danger to personnel intoxicated on PCP. In certain areas of these settings the hazard potential to co-workers and the public is second to none.

## Community Drug Treatment Programs

Most established programs for treating drug abuse focus on users of alcohol or heroin and other narcotics or on the emerging multiple

drug users. PCP is a wholly different problem. Administrators **81**
need to recognize that their traditional programs may not only be
ineffective in treating PCPers, but also may exacerbate their
problems.

In the past, many drug abusers not exposed to PCP were managed confrontively. The approach was firm yet supportive, with
much physical contact. Heroin users, for example, in a residential
treatment program often must go through major physical and emotional changes that to an outsider seem degrading. The rationale for
this approach is that heroin users need to develop coping skills in a
highly structured environment. Before heroin users can be rehabili-
tated, all the drug-related defense mechanisms essential to the heroin lifestyle must be broken down. As a result, highly confrontive,
attack-oriented therapy has become the basic model of treatment.

PCP does not fit this traditional picture. Since PCPers have
fragile egos that need support, attack therapy early in treatment is
counterproductive. In addition, the treatment picture is complicated by the retention of PCP in the body. At least thirty days
should pass before attack therapy is attempted. In fact, treatable
PCPers often need several months of recovery before effective
therapy can begin.

Community drug treatment personnel must adjust to PCP and
rise to its unique challenges. First, they must learn how to recognize PCPers. Further, since drug treatment personnel have relied on
their personal and working experience, they must often adapt to
handle PCP.

The survival of many drug treatment programs will depend on
the ability of their personnel to make the transition from other drug
problems to PCP. Restructuring these programs to meet the needs
of PCPers requires changes in staffing, setting, and management
procedures.

## Staffing

The first change all staffers must make is to shift their style from
confrontive to supportive. This change is of paramount importance.

Staffers also need to realize that whatever the circumstance under
which PCPers arrive, the drug is probably still in their systems.

**82**

Once it has been decided how best to handle a particular case, all the medical and first-aid procedures already discussed apply. Some PCPers will be kept in the treatment program after initial screening, and the program's goals should be to detoxify and habilitate them. Achieving these goals may require various changes in staffing and procedure. Whatever the specifics of such changes, several features are essential.

☐ The routine monitoring of PCPers for possible medical complications requires in-house physician services. The weight loss that accompanies chronic PCP abuse should be treated with dietary counseling.

☐ Ongoing psychological evaluation is required to detect shifts in mental status. Psychotherapy and medication should be available as needed to complete detoxification and to control severe depression and suicidal and aggressive behavior.

☐ Restraining aggressive PCPers and minimizing injury to clients and staff require a trained team of at least five staff members. The team should be available whenever a PCPer displays any of the four signs of toxicity discussed in Chapter 3 or has a history of violence. If too few staff members are present, measures should be established to obtain outside help from, for example, paramedics or police. Staff members should realize that the PCPer is being treated for a drug taken by choice and not out of ignorance or by accident.

## Setting

Handling PCPers may require changes in the intake environment. A crowded waiting room is inappropriate for PCPers, who need reduced stimulation. Hazards in the treatment setting, such as lamps, windows, chairs, and office equipment, should be identified and minimized. Since PCP clients are unpredictable and continuous monitoring may be impossible, all potential environmental hazards must be eliminated or controlled. Also, an alarm system may be needed to implement an emergency assistance plan for meeting a crisis created by a PCPer.

Management Procedures **83**

Handling PCPers well means following some basic guidelines.

☐ PCP abusers should be separated from other clients and monitored by personnel familiar with addiction and psychotic behavior.

☐ Confrontational models of treatment are inappropriate and potentially hazardous. Small supportive group models have been relatively effective in habilitating PCP clients.

☐ The prolonged effects of PCP on some clients may severely hamper the habilitation process. Certain PCPers will remain at the same level for several months.

☐ Persistent regressive behavior may signal reintoxication through recirculation or further use of the drug. Referral to medical or mental health services should be considered.

☐ Routine staff meetings should be held to review and revise treatment procedures and introduce new procedures gleaned from the experience and research of others.

☐ It is important to establish and maintain close working relationships with medical, mental health, and law enforcement personnel within the community.

## Community Mental Health

It has been our general experience that mental health personnel see three groups of PCPers. The first, and largest, group is the acute cases from emergency rooms or crisis services. Another group comprises those who come for help for what PCPers call "brain damage" or depression. The third group is made up of PCPers referred by concerned parents, teachers, drug treatment specialists, criminal justice personnel, and other human service providers.

All these PCPers are initially classified as inpatients or outpatients. However, since PCPers tend to go back to using the drug, outpatients may have to be admitted or readmitted immediately to an inpatient facility. We have seen PCPer inpatients who continued to use phencyclidine, getting the drug from friends or bringing it in with them. It is important to confiscate all drugs from the patient before admission and to screen all visitors.

## Inpatients

Most community mental health personnel are unfamiliar with nonopiate drug abuse. Many are not trained to care for such abusers and are reluctant to recognize or undertake the steps necessary for dealing with such patients, including PCPers (9).

Most PCPers admitted as inpatients are acutely psychotic. They are predominantly catatonic or violent; severe depression or suicidal behavior may also be evident. Caring for the PCPer entails several changes in the established procedures for treating psychiatric inpatients.

☐ PCPers who exhibit a blank stare and are noncommunicative or violent should be managed with sensory isolation in a quiet or se-clusion room. The room should be padded, have adjustable recessed lighting, and lack furniture or overhead fixtures that can be used to attempt suicide. Patients in this state require constant monitoring. They should not be approached or stimulated in any manner, since external stimulation can trigger violent behavior and necessitate aggressive intervention.

☐ Violent PCPers who present a danger to themselves or others should be placed in restraints by using the accumulative–body-weight method of control. Apply the restraints loosely to prevent acute myoglobinuria and acute kidney failure.

☐ If restraints do not calm the patient, medicate with diazepam. This is the drug of choice for all patients whose intoxication is evidenced by drug screening or by nystagmus, blank stare, or gait ataxia. Further details are given above in the discussion of emergency medical procedures.

# Prolonged Psychosis                                                          **85**

There appear to be two patient groups that are at risk from exposure to phencyclidines. Among those who become psychotic, approximately 25 percent return within a year for what appear to be typical symptoms of schizophrenic psychosis without further use of the drug (10,11). For some persons, sensitivity to the phencyclidines is immediate, whereas other PCPers generally display these symptoms only after chronic use. However, long-term psychosis may remit within each of these groups.

Recovery from long-term PCP psychosis involves three phases.

*Orientation.* Psychotic patients should be brought through a progressive orientation from isolation to appropriate social interaction. Once the patient appears normal, he or she is placed in a ward for a short time. If the assigned staff member observes any regression, the patient is taken back to the quiet or seclusion room. This process is repeated until the patient can handle the ward situation.

Patients often calm themselves by wrapping their bodies in a blanket. The patient should slowly be encouraged to take part in group activities. Ward situations that threaten overstimulation must be avoided, as confrontive techniques should be. The patient's acceptance of the social milieu of the ward is the first step toward integration.

*Integration.* Normally patients take five to twenty-one days after the onset of PCP-induced psychosis to return to their premorbid state. Although they may suddenly appear to be "normal," they commonly regress to the psychotic state. However, once their orientation is stable and continuously lucid, they can be integrated into the community.

The treatment staff must deal with the patients' potential for suicide and aggression. Commonly, patients ask "Why am I here?" and "Am I crazy?" Whenever possible, inform patients of how they were hospitalized and inform them of the past and present treatment plan. This reduces the patients' level of anxiety and sets the stage for habilitation. Some professionals have found video tapes of patients during acute hospitalization or in treatment helpful in convincing PCPers of their former behavior. However, this technique violates laws regarding informed consent and could have negative clinical ramifications.

Supportive individual and group therapy can be begun at this point. Time should be devoted to educating patients on the immediate and long-term effects of PCP intoxication.

*Habilitation.* The first prerequisite to habilitation is involving the family or significant others in treatment. They can help the patient over the transition from integration to habilitation. Shortly before discharge, the appropriate drug treatment personnel should contact PCP patients to develop a follow-up treatment plan in conjunction with mental health services.

## Outpatients

Most outpatients are inpatient referrals and PCPers in the confused state. Patients without recent medical records should be examined physically before treatment begins.

A number of concerns should be dealt with before a PCP outpatient program is established. The first is the staff's commitment to treating PCPers. Like many drug abusers, PCPers often progress little over a long time, even when all the program's resources are committed. PCPers are particularly resistant to intervention and often recycle through treatment programs.

Another concern is the staff's willingness to call for help when it is needed. Also, when a patient decompensates, the staff should consider hospitalization.

Finally, drug screening, medication, and therapeutic drug monitoring are needed. Since most PCP patients are polydrug abusers, they should be screened for both phencyclidines and other drugs. Mental health programs with budgetary constraints can make random screens of routinely collected samples. Urine, for example, can be pooled for analysis.

Managing ambulatory PCP patients requires clinical training and experience in treating violent and psychotic behavior. Adequate staffing and the emergency procedures developed for psychotic patients generally apply to PCPers. One difference is that as many as five staff members should be available to restrain violent PCPers.

Patients displaying nystagmus, gait ataxia, blank stare, muscle rigidity, and a lack of communication have ingested PCP recently. With such patients, the phenothiazines are contraindicated. Phenothiazines may be used, though, to control the antisocial behavior of patients who are no longer PCP toxic (as indicated by a lack of physical or toxicological findings). It has been suggested that tricyclic antidepressants may help severely depressed patients, but prescribing such drugs to patients depressed because of PCP is risky. Overdoses of tricyclic antidepressants cause any number of major problems, including arrhythmias, seizures, and hypotension, and they can be used to commit suicide. They should, therefore, be given only to patients with "endogenous type" depressions and not to those who are suicidal and unpredictably depressed.

All outpatients should be instructed to consume large amounts of cranberry juice and ascorbic acid. This acidifies the urine and, as we discussed earlier, it may help decrease PCP blood levels and speed recovery. Orange juice makes the urine basic and should not be used.

Generally, the same guidelines hold for inpatients and outpatients. As patients improve, psychotherapy should be used to address the underlying motivations related to drug abuse and to improve their quality of life.

## Reducing PCP Hazards in High-Risk Settings

Certain recreational and educational settings, military transport and weapons systems, and industrial environments present unusual risks to PCPers and bystanders. Each of these situations is different, but they all share common characteristics. The guidelines that follow serve to outline a systematic analysis for determining risk, so that those familiar with specific situations can undertake the measures best suited to their areas.

☐ Identify the most hazardous locations, such as laboratories, swimming pools, test ranges, machinery, radioactive systems, and aircraft maintenance.

☐  Determine the worst possible situation that could result from PCP intoxication.

☐  Determine what resources are needed and how they can be employed to meet that worst possible situation (e.g., turning off the power or fuel supply, isolating the PCPer, evacuating the area, or turning on fire-extinguishing equipment).

☐  Establish clear policies related to the use of PCP by individuals in high-risk areas.

With this groundwork laid, measures necessary for the specific needs of a particular setting can be taken.

## Summary

The general guidelines for managing PCPers are to use extreme caution, remove all hazards from the environment (particularly cars, weapons, and water), reduce all stimulation to the PCPer, and know your local resources.

Law enforcement officers need to recognize the telltale signs of PCP intoxication and to understand that traditional methods of control do not work on PCPers. Whenever PCP is suspected, officers should call for help immediately, wait the situation out if possible, use the accumulative–body-weight procedure when it is necessary to gain control of a PCPer, transport PCPers in restraints in an ambulance or squad car, clear PCPers medically, and monitor them constantly even when they appear cooperative.

Seizing and taking down a PCP laboratory involve considerable danger because of the toxic nature of the chemicals and the ever-present danger of fire and explosion. The operation requires an understanding of the hazards, proper personnel (including criminalists, paramedics, and firefighters), and adherence to basic safety precautions.

Emergency medical treatment of PCP intoxication is symptomatic. PCPers in the confused state should be kept quiet and secluded and be constantly monitored. Agitated PCPers should first be quieted and secluded. If this does not calm them, diazepam should **89** be used. If this too fails, restraints are the next step. Comatose PCPers are a medical emergency requiring gastric aspiration and lavage, medication, and continuous monitoring of vital signs. Prolonged comatose patients are handled in much the same way. Ion trapping—acidification treatment to speed the elimination of PCP remains experimental. Care should be taken not to discharge PCPers too soon and to be sure that their home environment presents no dangers to themselves or to their families. Discharged PCPers should be referred to the appropriate drug treatment and mental health professionals.

PCPers do not fit the traditional community drug treatment model. Changes must be made to adapt to their needs. Staffers must be supportive instead of confrontive, ready to monitor PCPers constantly, and trained to handle violent and aggressive PCPers. Hazards have to be eliminated from treatment settings, and new management procedures must be established.

Community mental health personnel see PCPers as both inpatients and outpatients. Inpatients are usually acutely psychotic. They need to be monitored and secluded, and, if violent, restrained or medicated. In cases of prolonged psychosis, PCPers need to be led from orientation to integration to habilitation. Treating outpatient PCPers demands strong staff commitment despite the poor payoff, a willingness to call for help, drug screening and medication as needed, and clinical training in handling violent patients.

The dangers from PCP intoxication in high-risk settings can be reduced by analyzing the dangers of the setting and taking the necessary precautions.

**90** **PART III** CHAPTER 5

PREVENTING LITIGATING
PCP THE
ABUSE PCPer

Criminal acts associated with intoxication from PCP and other **91** phencyclidines have created a serious problem for the courts. Few members of the judicial system are familiar with the unique properties of this new family of drugs and the major points that need to be established in the litigation of PCP-related criminal acts. This chapter details the law applying to the manufacture, sale, possession, and use of PCP, reviews the nature of criminal law as it applies to PCP, and examines how PCP intoxication can influence criminal proceedings.

## PCP in the Law

The federal and state laws that apply to the manufacture, sale, possession, and use of PCP are based primarily on the Controlled Substances Act, which classifies drugs into five groups, ranging from most to least dangerous. The first group of drugs, called Schedule I, includes such well-known hazardous substances as heroin and LSD. PCP is classified in Schedule II, which includes substances that have a high potential for abuse and may lead to severe psychological or physical dependence but have a restricted but acceptable medical use in the United States.

It is our opinion that PCP should be reclassified to Schedule I. This change would raise the penalty for manufacture and sale from five to fifteen years, adding a badly needed deterrent. Given the recent upsurge in the abuse of other phencyclidines, all the PCP analogs should also be added to Schedule I. The major obstacle to this move, unfortunately, is the continued medical use of Ketamine, which limits the control of the other phencyclidines. The legal manufacture of phencyclidines contributes to the expansion of this new drug problem and undermines the activities of the criminal justice system.

Attempts have been made to control PCP manufacture indirectly by restricting the possession of the immediate precursors needed to make piperidine or cyclohexanone and of piperidine, cyclohexanone, or a combination of both in order to make PCP. These restrictions do work some benefit, but they also make these products more scarce, increasing their price and profits and raising the incentive to manufacture them.

# 92    PCP and Criminality

Making or possessing PCP is only the beginning of the criminality associated with PCP. PCP affects behavior profoundly, even tragically, and the behavior of PCPers often makes them the focus of criminal action.

## The Nature of Criminal Law

The oldest known codification of criminal law dates back 2000 years to the Babylonian king Hammurabi, who formalized a strict and simple interpretation of "an eye for an eye, a tooth for a tooth." Someone who took the life or limb of another suffered the same penalty in return. Result determined punishment. The law ignored both the degree of fault and the intent of the wrongdoer. Killing was killing, whether the killer took life accidentally or intentionally.

Over the centuries this early legal system changed to take into account the intent of the individual's act. Intent is now as important as conduct. Our current system requires that the responsibility for an act be determined by whether the prescribed conduct coincides with the requisite mental state or intent (1).

Thus, for example, unlawful killing is divided into a number of crimes. First degree murder entails the willful, deliberate, and premeditated killing of another, or, in some states, the accidental or intentional killing of another during a violent felony like arson, rape, or robbery — what is called felony murder. To be liable for first degree murder, the killer must intend to kill, must have formed that intent as the result of a careful and rational weighing of the considerations for and against the killing, and must have considered and decided before the actual killing. Second degree murder entails killing another with malice aforethought, but without the willfulness, deliberation, or premeditation of first degree murder. Manslaughter involves the killing of another without malice aforethought; it may be voluntary, if the killing was intended, or accidental, if it was not. Thus the law takes a given act — the killing of another human — and determines the severity of the crime by assaying the mental status of the killer.

As a result, the law now generally recognizes that certain indi- **93** viduals, by reason of insanity or mental incapacity (legally, diminished capacity), do not have the requisite mental state and that their criminal responsibility is limited or removed. By extension, a defendant must be able to exercise rational intellect and free will to make a voluntary confession.

Here PCP complicates this seemingly clear picture. Besides manufacturing and possessing, PCP has been involved in such crimes as driving under the influence, robbery and burglary, arson, rape, child endangering, and homicide. Drug intoxication, even when it is voluntary, may be sufficient cause to suppress a defendant's confession or to allow a defense of diminished capacity.

## PCP, Insanity, and the Diminished Capacity Defense

Because of the unique and predictably unpredictable nature of PCP intoxication, interpretation of the law regarding criminal responsibility is problematic. The majority of PCP-related cases involving criminal acts are litigated by an insanity or diminished capacity defense. The American Law Institute Test for insanity is (2):

A person is not responsible for criminal conduct if at the time of such conduct as a result of mental disease or defect he lacks the substantial capacity either to appreciate the criminality of his conduct or to conform his conduct to the requirements of the law.

Insanity from PCP toxicity arises when the person who has committed the crime appears severely disabled.

Case #2005.

A thirty-year-old male, who had been using PCP for several months, began dancing, chanting, and painting the number 7 on his furniture and children. He was subsequently taken to a county psychiatric facility for commitment. After a brief period of observation, he was released since there was no evidence of mental disease during that time. A couple of hours later he appeared at his mother's house nude. He proceeded to stab his two-year-old son to death and severely cut his mother.

Persistent psychosis induced by PCP intoxication prevents this man from understanding the nature of the charges or from cooperating with defense counsel. He has not been brought to trial.

The insanity defense requires proof of a settled condition, which may come and go, that deprives the individual of the ability to control his or her behavior freely and intelligently. This condition is beyond that produced by recent use of PCP (3):

> While phencyclidine-induced psychosis may result from usage of the drug on one occasion only, it may be argued that the prolonged duration of the psychotic episode makes the mental effect produced by ingestion of the drug more akin to insanity than to the acute condition produced by voluntary intoxication. Since all users of the drug do not suffer such a reaction from ingesting even a large quantity of PCP, it can be argued further that the drug merely unmasks a preexisting psychopathology and is not the underlying cause of the aberrational mental state. Relying on these arguments, counsel may attempt to circumvent the limitations of the voluntary intoxication defense.

The diminished capacity defense of criminal acts committed by someone under the influence of PCP assumes that the drug caused an abnormal physical or mental condition. The PCP-induced condition must prevent the defendant from, in the language of the law, "maturely and meaningfully premeditating, deliberating, and reflecting upon the gravity of the contemplated act."

The diminished capacity defense applies traditionally to cases that require proof of specific intent; generally it is not accepted as a defense to crimes of general intent. Because PCP can affect perception, it may affect one's ability to form specific intent, since such intent requires a high level of mental functioning. Therefore, diminished capacity is an appropriate defense when it can be shown that the criminal act was committed under the influence of PCP, which caused a mental condition impairing the individual's ability to "maturely and meaningfully premeditate, deliberate, and reflect upon the gravity of the contemplated act."

Generally juries do not go out of their way to accept a defense of insanity or diminished capacity based on PCP intoxication. It has been our experience that in a trial for first degree murder with convincing evidence, a verdict of second degree murder should occasionally be expected. With the sentiment growing among juries that criminals should be jailed rather than treated, a verdict of voluntary manslaughter is unlikely.

Violent acts associated with PCP intoxication have been divided into four categories (4). Type I acts, including violent criminal offenses or conscious suicide activities, are ". . . reality-oriented, goal-directed violence in individuals with reasonably coherent thought processes and intact memory and impulse control . . ." (4). Type II acts include " . . . unexpected, impulsive violence in persons with diminished internal controls and decreased reality orientation . . ." (4). Such compulsive criminal and suicidal acts are often recalled with mildly impaired mental functioning. Type III acts can be classified as " . . . unexpected violence, often directed toward some bizarre or idiosyncratic personal goal, usually independent of reality goals and often including some element of stereotyped repetitive action and primitive sadistic behavior" (4). The ability to coordinate movements remains intact; however, the PCPer usually is unable to recall the incident and is most likely in the uncommunicative agitated state. Type IV acts encompass " . . . severe disorganized psychotic or organic agitation, with chaotic, incoordinated violent behavior" (4).

This classification scheme, supported by our clinical and court experiences, should prove helpful in litigating PCP related acts.

## PCP and First Degree Murder

The number of first degree murder cases in which PCP intoxication is used as the defense is alarming. The litigation of these cases is subject to a broad range of interpretation based largely on the available evidence and the expert witnesses' familiarity with the unique properties of the phencyclidines.

A defense based on PCP intoxication is easiest to conduct when the defendant is apprehended immediately or soon after the crime, when the defendant has a urine level pH-specific for PCP, and when eyewitnesses observe the signs of PCP intoxication. If the defendant is apprehended well after the crime, the difficulty of developing a PCP defense increases, getting harder the more time it took to find and arrest the defendant.

## Case #2231.

A thirty-year-old male with a long history of drug abuse starting at age thirteen was riding on the back of a motorcycle with a friend after smoking a PCP joint. The motorcycle broke down in a residential area. The defendant walked to a nearby house to use the phone to call a relative for assistance. An elderly man let the defendant in his house to make the telephone call. The defendant proceeded to murder the man with a knife taken from the kitchen. Before leaving, he took some pennies from the man's bedroom even though the victim had $200 in his shirt pocket. The defendant was apprehended several days later, found guilty of first degree murder, and given the death penalty.

Since defense counsel had no toxicological findings nor independent eyewitnesses, a good defense was hard to establish. The prosecutor, on the other hand, raised serious doubts in the minds of the jurors about whether the defendant had actually taken PCP and, if he had, whether the dose was enough to keep him from appreciating the consequences of his acts.

In cases such as this, toxicological findings are crucial, but they are by no means unequivocal. In all cases they bear careful study for error. It has been our experience that laboratory results are not always accurate. In one case of obvious drug intoxication verified by recordings made during police interrogation, the police crime laboratory reported totally negative findings for the common drugs of abuse from blood and urine samples. Subsequently, an independent toxicologist using gas chromatography/mass spectrometry found a near lethal concentration of secobarbital, as well as methaqualone, diazepam, and PCP.

Body fluid samples may be tested for PCP for a long while after they are collected. A study to determine the stability of PCP in forty-five samples of stored blood preserved with sodium fluoride and potassium oxalate found no changes in PCP concentrations for

up to eighteen months (5). We have been involved in cases where **97**
defendants' blood and urine were successfully analyzed for PCP as
long as one year after the samples were taken. Thus, in questionable
cases, rechecking can be worthwhile.

## PCP and Second Degree Murder

In some states, the seller of an illicit drug that causes the death of a
buyer can be found guilty of second degree murder.

## Case #2101.

Two sisters in their early twenties, after sharing a PCP joint and wine,
climbed into a hot tub to "enjoy the high." A few minutes later, one of the
young women was discovered by the other face down in the water. Upon
searching the house of the person who had sold them the PCP, police found
a jar of parsley, cigarette papers, and a PCP joint. The seller was arrested
and subsequently found guilty of second degree murder.

## Driving Under the Influence

One of the most common PCP-related criminal acts is driving
under the influence. This case is typical.

## Case #2019.

A fifty-year-old produce truck driver was forced to stop by opposing traffic as he attempted to enter a freeway offramp in the wrong direction. The
arresting officer reported the man's eyes were bloodshot and his speech

thick. It was difficult for the man to remove his driver's license from his wallet and get out of his vehicle. He staggered through the Field Sobriety Test. He was not able to stand on one foot without stumbling. His blood contained 10 ng/ml of PCP with no other drugs present.

Both behavior following the incident and blood test confirmed PCP intoxication, which the defendant did not contest.

Driving under the influence of PCP may well have contributed to a sudden rise in automobile accidents in several metropolitan areas. The distorted perceptions caused by the drug lead to arrests and fatalities.

## Case #2126.

A male in his twenties, with 0.4 mcg/ml of PCP in his urine, drove down the wrong side of a street in a business district in southern California. At approximately 70 miles per hour, his vehicle jumped the curb and drove through the wall of a sandwich shop, killing three women.

The driver was prosecuted for vehicular manslaughter. The case, which we were involved in, evidences some of the complications of PCP-related criminal trials. The defendant claimed that he became unconscious "while driving at the speed limit from straining to sing a high note." However, he was seen immediately after the accident staggering and speaking in a slurred manner, signs of PCP intoxication. Examination in an emergency room revealed no evidence of head trauma to account for the postaccident behavior or the unconsciousness alleged to have caused the collision. Despite the PCP level of 0.4 mcg/ml in the urine, no PCP appeared in the blood.

The defense was based on unconsciousness from trying to hit a high note. The expert witness for the defense claimed that since no PCP was detected in the defendant's blood, the defendant was not under the drug's influence. He also stated that he knew of no published reports on blood and urine levels of PCP related to car accidents.

We testified to the contrary for the prosecution. We concluded that the level of PCP in the urine and the defendant's aberrant behavior after the accident showed that PCP caused the erratic driving leading to the accident. In support, we presented data on the urine levels typical of chronic PCPers, death victims, and drivers under the influence (6,7,8).

**99**

### PCP Urine Levels

| Group | Range (mcg/ml) |
|---|---|
| Chronic users | 0.03–10.5 |
| Death victims | 0.05–330.0 |
| Drivers under the influence | 0.19–21.2 |

The bottom range in each of these groups lies below the defendant's 0.4 mcg/ml; in short, the defendant had more than enough PCP in him to cause the accident. Indeed, our investigations have uncovered deaths from behavioral toxicity at PCP urine levels as low as 0.05 mcg/ml. As to the apparent absence of PCP in the defendant's blood, we found that the method of analysis used was inadequate because of its limited sensitivity. Also, we cited several cases from the literature that related PCP levels to driving violations.

The defendant was found guilty on all counts. It could not be submitted as evidence at the trial, but the defendant had recently been cited for two moving violations and a joint wrapped in foil and apparently containing PCP was found in his car at the time of the accident.

In another driving-under-the-influence case, the prosecution was unable to convince the jury of significant PCP intoxication in the absence of quantitative toxicological evidence. Therefore, it is not sufficient to have merely a positive urine for PCP. The amount of PCP in the urine and the pH of that urine at the time it was taken are essential prerequisites to a successful prosecution.

# 100    The Expert Witness in PCP Cases

The expert witness is often the key to successful prosecution or defense of a PCP-related proceeding. To add to a legal effort, an expert witness must be able both to verify that the defendant was intoxicated on phencyclidine and to describe the effects of the drug on the defendant. Ideally, the expert should have experience in clinical research on, and the treatment of, the effects of phencyclidines on humans.

Still, even under the best of circumstances, the expert witness is in a difficult position. Litigation of PCP cases is inconsistent and confusing. Part of the cause for this state of affairs is the idiosyncratic effects PCP has on different people. In addition, appropriate medical-legal definitions of intoxication, impaired mental function, diminished capacity, and insanity related to voluntary PCP intoxication have yet to be determined. Such issues as differences in the sensitivity and specificity of analytical tests, the relationship between toxicological findings and mental status, inconsistent medical and legal nomenclature, unqualified expert witnesses, and variability in the legal process contribute to the vast confusion surrounding PCP cases. All too often the expert witness is asked to give a black or white response to a question whose true answer lies in the gray area somewhere in between.

## Prerequisites to Litigation

Preparing to prosecute or defend in a PCP case demands attention to details. Those details fall into several main areas.

### Toxicology

The defendant's body fluids should be screened quantitatively and qualitatively for the phencyclidines and other commonly abused drugs, including alcohol. To enable proper interpretation of PCP levels in urine, the pH of the urine should also be determined immediately. Gas chromatography/mass spectrometry should be used to test for phencyclidines, and the credentials of the personnel conducting the analytic tests and the methods they use should be documented.

## Physical and Neurological Examination

The defendant should be given a complete physical and neurological examination immediately, and all findings, both positive and negative, should be recorded.

## Psychological Assessment

The defendant's psychological status should be determined through a drug-use history, family history, educational history, psychiatric history, and psychometric/projective testing, including actual data.

## Psychiatric Assessment

A history of the defendant's childhood, adolescence, and so forth should be obtained, in addition to family history, illness survey, mental status examination, and a psychiatric diagnosis and recommendations.

## Relevant Documentation

To aid the expert witness, all relevant documentary evidence should be gathered and cataloged. This evidence will include police records, preliminary transcripts, statements of witnesses, de-

**102**

fendant's statement (preferably on audio or video tape), booking information, information on the conduct and condition of the defendant in custody, school records, prior probation and presentencing reports, employment records, military service records, prison records, medical or psychiatric records, and the results and methods of all laboratory tests.

## Summary

PCP belongs to Schedule II on the Controlled Substances Act. Changing the drug's status to Schedule I would increase penalties and add to the deterrent.

PCP affects the application of criminal law because it compromises a clear understanding of the criminal's intent at the time the crime is committed. Psychosis from chronic PCP intoxication may lead to an insanity defense, and acute PCP intoxication may lead to a diminished capacity defense. In first degree murder cases, both defenses rest on positive toxicological findings and eyewitness testimony to the defendant's bizarre behavior. In some states, selling a drug that proves lethal to the buyer constitutes second degree murder. Driving under the influence is a common PCP-related crime.

PCP cases often depend on expert witnesses, who must verify PCP intoxication and describe the drug's effects. Their role is made more difficult by the legal inconsistencies surrounding PCP and the lack of clear-cut answers.

Proper litigation of PCP cases demands attention to toxicology, physical and neurological examination, psychological and psychiatric assessment of the defendant, and all relevant documentation.

# CHAPTER 6          103

## COMMUNITY
## ACTION
## TO STOP
## PCP ABUSE

To recognize and manage PCPers, coordination between community human service providers is essential. However, most such professionals have traditionally been trained and reinforced to work individually and make decisions on their own. Most human problems, including drug abuse, cross disciplinary boundaries, and their solution, therefore, requires input from each of those disciplines. Drug abuse is a prime example; it is both the cause and the symptom of much human suffering. Our approach to it, though, has been reductionist and simplistic. Emphasis is still laid on drugs as causes instead of symptoms, and the Harrison Act of 1914 transfers responsibility for solving drug abuse problems from individuals and health professionals to the government. This approach falls well short. Health personnel realize that trying to reduce drug abuse in a drug-oriented culture by outlawing drugs alone is like trying to prevent tooth decay by enacting a prohibition on candy. To respond realistically to the problem, we must respond collectively to the whole person with an emphasis on the forces that cause people to rely on drugs instead of each other. An essential prerequisite to this collective response is educating human service providers to recognize and manage drug abuse through a holistic approach — a network.

The network design detailed in this chapter has proved effective in setting and attaining community goals on PCP abuse. Here we present an outline of the basics. The ultimate design and make-up of a given local network will depend on local needs, resources, financial and political considerations, and other related community factors.

## Multicultural Issues

Basic to the building of a community network is an understanding of the multicultural dimensions of the PCP problem. Over the past decade, human service providers have come to realize that they must interpret drug abuse from the perspectives of many cultures. The unique properties of PCP and its use by youth from all ethnic groups in the United States require a better understanding of cultural diversity — which implies sensitivity to race, religion, sex, language, socioeconomic status, interests, geographic origin, and history. Taking a multicultural view of PCP means becoming aware of the characteristics unique to a culture that affect the prevention and prevalence of PCP abuse and the management and habilitation of PCPers.

The success of human service providers dealing with minority PCPers depends largely on whether they are bilingual and bicultural. Professionals must be particularly careful not to perceive PCPers from one culture through the values and goals of their own culture. They must recognize and understand the PCPer's life in total, accounting for those dilemmas created by those persons in the PCPer's life who do admit to cultural pluralism and who penalize minority people for not adhering to some fictional standard of the "model" American. PCP workers in a multicultural setting must believe that the wholeness of our society springs from the unique contributions of each of its diverse parts.

PCP-abuse professionals must face the principal issue that the perspectives on abusing drugs, particularly PCP, differ significantly among ethnic groups. This raises a further issue: what are the sound and meaningful alternatives to PCP abuse? For example, gangs often provide a way for youth to release anger and frustration, and drugs have traditionally played an important role in gang violence. Certain properties of PCP — disinhibition, high suggestibility, and anesthesia — have made PCP popular among gangs. By the same token, gang members who oppose violence or are afraid may use PCP as a way of avoiding criminal acts or summoning up the courage they lack.

To halt their abuse, PCPers have to be directed from self-destructive activities to self-improvement. The alternatives human service providers present to PCPers must be relevant ways of generating positive self-concepts and pride in the PCPers' culture and community.

## Building a Network

The network strategy has grown out of the inadequacy of old answers for the new problems presented by PCP.

**106**   A Bit of Background

The linking of criminal justice and community drug treatment personnel in both training and cooperation has been problematic, in part because ex-offenders commonly work in drug treatment. This difficult situation has been relieved somewhat by the movement toward free clinics and other modalities of prevention and intervention. Crisis and walk-in centers have grown rapidly, in part because official agencies have not responded well to drug abusers.

To overcome this division among agencies, we embarked a few years back on an interdisciplinary training effort that brought together human service providers who traditionally did not interact in response to the growing PCP problem. The basis for this state-funded project was that the management problems presented by PCP abuse were best met when human service providers were willing to enter into dialogue. For example, law enforcement personnel, who were the first to see the fright and horror of the PCP problem, were frustrated over the uselessness of their traditional methods of control, and that frustration drove them to open channels of communication with professionals in drug treatment. Such efforts were the beginning of the network strategy we have since developed.

The most enlightened theory points out that change must come from both the top down and the bottom up. That is, those who work at the bottom with PCPers must perceive the need for, and actively participate in, the linking with top-down, or administrative, support. This rationale has stood the acid test in California, and from our training project many county networks for community action on the PCP problem have arisen.

Building a Network

The community action process that mobilizes resources is the key to building a network successfully. The components that must be linked in the network are community service resources (i.e., human service providers) and those requiring service (i.e., youth and parents).

## The Network Model

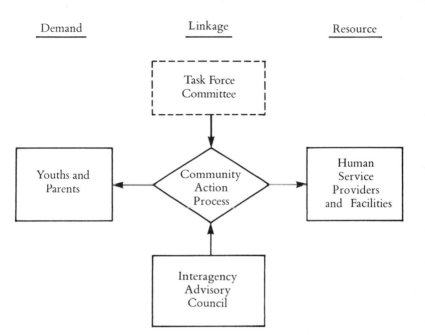

This network model represents a demand-linkage-resource strategy, which arises from a communitywide need for an interdisciplinary response to the PCP problem. The community action process begins by defining the demand for services and then the resources required to satisfy that demand.

In our experience, the better linked human service providers are to others who share the same concerns and convictions about PCP abuse, the better able they are to start the action process. The task force committee should be composed of such a representative group of concerned providers as the prime movers of the community action process.

**Community Action Process**

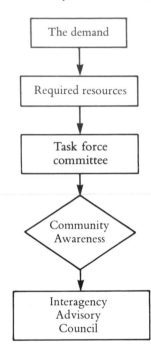

The synthesizing of human service providers, essential for net-working, can be achieved through community awareness activities. One way of bringing human service providers to appreciate the nature of PCP abuse is for the task force to hold a communitywide hearing on the PCP problem. The hearing establishes the need for the next step — an activity or event to provide information about PCP abuse.

This informational activity — conference, workshop, or forum — should culminate in the formation of an interagency advisory group that represents the community agencies that provide human services related to PCP abuse. This activity identifies the community's needs related to PCP abuse, establishes goals, and starts action planning.

## Components of the Network **109**

With this basic outline of the network in mind, let's look closely at its basic elements.

## Demand for Services

Those in need of services related to PCP abuse are primarily youth and parents. Numbered among the youth are PCPers, those at risk, and those not yet exposed to illicit drugs. Parents and parents of prospective PCPers are also included in this group.

One way of defining the demand for PCP-related services is to conduct a survey to determine the nature and extent of the problem within the community. Law enforcement, emergency medicine, drug treatment, and mental health services are essential sources of information about the problem in the local community. Chapter 1 identifies other sources.

## Resources

Analyzing survey results will reveal at least the major resources required to meet the local demand for PCP abuse services. These results are important even if PCP is not yet a major problem in the community. Communities that have conducted surveys before PCP arrived in their locale have been able to compare their findings with the experiences of communities already beset by the PCP problem and thus have been able to forecast what might happen. A clear understanding of the problem and early preparation for it appear to dampen the escalation of the PCP problem once it begins.

## Task Force Committee

The interdisciplinary task force should comprise professionals who provide services normally needed by PCPers (e.g., law enforcement, community mental health, emergency medicine, etc.). Participation should be at each individual's choice. Often the committee is responsible for conducting the survey to determine the demand for services, but in some communities drug abuse specialists perform this task. However the survey is done, the committee's course of action depends on its findings. The committee's major tasks are to collect information, plan and hold a communitywide hearing on PCP abuse, and conduct a community awareness activity that leads to establishing an interagency advisory council on the abuse of PCP and related drugs. Many communities already have such a council. If so, new consideration should be given to its membership, which may need to be expanded to include additional community provider groups affected by PCP abuse. Also, public officials can be included to generate interest and commitment to the community action process.

If the task force is to succeed, the membership, size, and leadership of the committee must be right. The nature of the community should be considered in forming the task force committee. Both providers and consumers of service should be included, with a balance of men and women selected to represent the ethnic, age, and socioeconomic characteristics of the community.

The committee has fulfilled its catalytic function in facilitating the community action process once a task-oriented interagency advisory council is established. The council's prime function is to establish and maintain the network.

## Community Awareness

Public awareness activity related to PCP abuse is the vehicle to bring the community together to initiate a plan for networking, expanding, improving, and evaluating PCP abuse services. The activity provides awareness of PCP abuse and initiates the networking needed for activities and community services.

The information activity can take any of a variety of forms and forums — public films, like those listed in the appendix, an official hearing, or a town meeting, for example — and its exact nature should be chosen to best fit the nature and idiosyncracies of the

particular community. Whatever its form, the activity should in-   **111**
clude several aspects of PCP abuse:

☐   Nature and extent of PCP abuse in the community
☐   An orientation to PCP abuse through
     an understanding of what PCP is and what it does
     the patterns of PCP abuse
     the impact of PCPers on the community
☐   Recognizing and managing PCPers in
     the criminal justice system
     medicine and mental health
     educational and religious institutions
     drug treatment programs
     recreation programs
     industry
☐   Alternative recreational activities in the community
☐   Resource sharing and interagency networking
☐   Action planning and the establishing of an interagency advisory
    council
☐   The role of unemployment and local economic depression in es-
    calating drug abuse among youth.

    This mutual awareness activity allows knowledge and perspec-
tives on local PCP abuse to be shared. Identifying common needs
related to PCP abuse and creating communication channels among
agencies to meet those needs penetrate the barriers to networking.
The activity leads ultimately to the setting up of an interagency
advisory council. Several factors are critical in establishing a successful council:

☐   Realistic and acceptable goals
☐   Appropriate and capable membership
☐   Effective leadership
☐   Mutual support

**112**     Interagency Advisory Council

How well the network succeeds in meeting local needs arising from the abuse of PCP and related drugs depends on how well the council maintains dialogue among the various human services. That dialogue should include areas peculiar to the abuse of PCP:

☐     Modification of traditional drug treatment approaches to PCP abuse
☐     Habilitation strategies for chronic PCPers requiring long-term care
☐     Multicultural difference in the demand for PCP abuse services
☐     Activities designed to prevent PCP abuse and promote public safety
☐     Dissemination of new information on the recognition, management, and prevention of PCP abuse

Never has the opportunity been greater for establishing a community network for drug abuse. The unique characteristics of PCP abuse create optimal conditions for all the activities essential to community network building, problem solving, and action planning. In this period of dwindling resources, the burden of responsibility for making the network a viable alternative to the usual fragmented efforts rests with each human service provider and each council member. There is no substitute for dedication. Already community networks have cut the costs of PCP abuse for PCPers, the community, and others.

Still, networks, good as they are, are not the ultimate answer. The real solution lies in prevention.

## Prevention: Our Best Hope for the Future

If we wish to survive our own chemical creations, we must become aware of our drug-oriented culture in order not to be unconsciously swayed by it. American society has entered a new age of drug abuse, and the ultimate challenge of the twenty-first century is to **113** survive ourselves. Chemical preparations are now available to solve every problem. Consumers have been conditioned to cope with stress with over-the-counter preparations — better living through chemistry, so to speak. That attitude is just a stone's throw from full-blown drug abuse. And the abundant and sophisticated technology that manufactures all those drugs has filtered down into the illicit markets. PCP, indeed, is the first of the synthetic drugs made easily from readily available ingredients at low cost and with little technical knowledge or specialized equipment.

The polydrug nature of PCP abuse is also reinforced by the common culture. Through self-administration, consumers may take one drug to combat the effects of another. Physicians themselves sometimes treat one drug problem with another drug, an occasionally necessary medical step that is also practiced by naive patients or youthful drug abusers, who have developed their own combinations of street drugs.

Each drug problem has its own identity or culture — marijuana and jazz musicians, alcohol and skid row, cocaine and the entertainment industry, for example. PCP appears to reinforce certain reactions of youth to the inequities of their daily lives. It is a new avenue of chemical escape, with the same shortcomings as all the other drugs that have promised the same sort of chemical solace.

The introduction of new drugs — affecting psychological functioning in unfamiliar ways — into the illicit drug scene is promoted by mass communication, the same prime mover of rapid culture change that feeds drug abuse. Contributing to this vicious circle are frustrations and stresses about having to do more with less in the face of an uncertain future.

Quantitatively, it is apparent that our civilization has advanced farther and faster than any before it. But from a qualitative perspective, one doubts just how real this progress is. In spite of all the miraculous achievements of medical science, the average number of years people live beyond forty is holding steady. The myriad effects of the stress we live with in our daily lives are fast becoming the scourge infectious disease once was. In this society, the chances are slim that one can have both success and good health. Unless we recognize this and take measures to lessen the demands for competition and to make success possible in the context of more healthful lifestyles, the frustrations of our youth will mount and drug abuse will grow apace.

PCP is not one drug problem. In a country so complex and technologically interwoven that it not only sends astronauts to the moon but also provides live TV coverage of the event, all drug problems are interwoven into an intricate fabric of human suffering, technology, and social and political institutions. Indeed, we cannot even look at PCP as a "problem" demanding a "solution." It is instead a dilemma best stopped before it begins. Our true hope for the future is preventing PCP abuse.

The reasons why people continuously seek drugs to alter their state of consciousness are as varied and complex as the people themselves. Therefore, the means of prevention must be just as varied and complex—which is a way of saying that there is no right way or wrong way. All approaches are needed so long as they promote a positive self-image and do not become part of the problem. No matter what, some people will always use or abuse drugs and youth in particular will experiment with them. As a result, we firmly believe that one should use, abuse, or experiment with drugs knowledgeably, not ignorantly. Therefore, any response to the PCP epidemic should include facts, both good and bad, about its use. Knowledge is power, and such power is central to controlling PCP abuse.

How a person responds to a drug depends on how that person views the drug, and that view is in part determined by social circumstance. Youths develop drug problems in part because they feel unable to take responsibility for life situations. The ability to take responsibility, reinforced by successful adult role models and early success that builds self-esteem, creates a sense of control, power, and focus on your life situation. Taking responsibility means not surrendering it to jails, mental institutions, or drugs. A well-developed sense of responsibility stands in the way of drug abuse. Therefore, it is the ultimate responsibility of parents, teachers, and human service providers to foster the concept that we are all responsible for ourselves.

The only dependency that promotes human potential is commitment to socially acceptable values. Everyone chooses whether to reject or accept family admonitions, religion, the culture, and the value of schooling or work. To rebel or accept is a choice. And to acknowledge the problem and solve it by applying chosen values is to accept the consequences of those values whether one likes it or not. This is the project to which we must all be committed as

human beings. The responsibility of those concerned about pre- **115**
venting drug abuse is to instruct youth about the importance, gravity, and power associated with having to choose.

Fostering such responsibility in youth requires a redefinition of
parenthood and education. Both of these nurturing processes must
take on a much broader meaning. Learning opportunities should be
lifelong, diverse, and individualized. Increasingly, multicultural
education will be essential to building a world community. In the
education process interdisciplinary problem solving should replace
"computermind" approaches to issues that lack yes-or-no, black-
and-white solutions. Youth should be encouraged to create alternatives to current practices that do not work.

PCP is fast becoming the ultimate drop-out drug among youth.
As with all drug abuse, the closer you get to the cause, the further
you are from the drug itself. To prevent continued PCP abuse we
must prepare youth to take responsibility for humanity's future. If
we are to survive ourselves, the "me first" orientation of personal
philosophy must yield to a "we first" concept of life.

## Summary

Recognizing and managing PCPers demands cooperation among
human service providers trained and used to working alone. The
complexity of the PCP problem requires a collective approach.

Dealing with PCP abuse means being sensitive to the multicultural nature of the drug problem. Both the problem and its solution
must be seen in terms relevant to particular ethnic communities.

The network strategy opens lines of communication and cooperation among agencies that traditionally have not worked together.
Networking requires a community action process that mobilizes
resources to meet needs.

The essentials of the network are the demand for services to treat
PCP abuse, community resources, a task force committee, activities designed to create community awareness of the PCP problem, and an interagency advisory council.

The best way to end PCP abuse is to stop it before it starts. Our society is beset with drug problems that are the offshoot of our dubious technological progress. Youthful abuse of PCP springs largely from a low sense of responsibility for life and feelings of being overwhelmed by a complex world. This basic motivation can best be overcome by parents and educators who seek to instill in young people a sense of the importance of choosing values.

**118 PART IV**

APPENDIXES

CHAPTER
REFERENCES

GLOSSARY

REFERRAL
AGENCIES LIST

BIBLIOGRAPHY

FILM LIST

PCP ABUSE
TRAINING
OUTLINE

## Chapter References                                    **119**

## Introduction

1. Burns, R. S.; Lerner, S. E.; Corrado, R.; James, S. H.; and Schnoll, S. H. "Phencyclidine — States of Acute Intoxication and Fatalities." *The Western Journal of Medicine* 123(5):348.

2. Burns, R. S., and Lerner, S. E. "Street PCP Use: Clinical Studies of the Acute and Chronic Intoxicated State." *Newsletter of the California Association of Toxicologists,* August 1975, pp. 32–59.

3. Burns, R. S., and Lerner, S. E. "The Phencyclidine Dilemma." *Newsletter of the California Society for the Treatment of Alcoholism and Other Drug Dependencies* 3(2):1–3.

4. Burns, R. S., and Lerner, S. E. "Phencyclidine: An Emerging Drug Problem." *Clinical Toxicology* 9(4):473–475.

5. Burns, R. S., and Lerner, S. E. "Perspectives: Acute Phencyclidine Intoxication." *Clinical Toxicology* 9(4):477–501.

6. Burns, R. S., and Lerner, S. E. "Perspectives: Acute Phencyclidine Intoxication (Revised)." *Proceedings of the Thirty-Eighth Annual Scientific Meeting, Committee on Problems of Drug Dependence.* Richmond, Va.: National Academy of Sciences, 1976, pp. 552–574.

7. Burns, R. S., and Lerner, S. E. "Management and Treatment of Acute Phencyclidine Intoxication." In P. E. Bourne, ed., *Acute Drug Abuse Emergencies: A Treatment Manual.* New York: Academic Press, 1976, pp. 297–305.

## Chapter 1

1. Burns, R. S., and Lerner, S. E. "Perspectives: Acute Phencyclidine Intoxication (revised)." *Proceedings of the Thirty-Eighth Annual Scientific Meeting, Committee on Problems of Drug Dependence.* Richmond, Va.: National Academy of Sciences, 1976, pp. 552–574.

2. Burns, R. S., and Lerner, S. E. "Management and Treatment of Acute Phencyclidine Intoxication." In P. E. Bourne, ed., *Acute*

**120**

*Drug Abuse Emergencies: A Treatment Manual.* New York: Academic Press, 1976, pp. 297– 305.

3. Rosen, A. "Case Report: Symptomatic Mania and Phencyclidine Abuse." *American Journal of Psychiatry* 136(1):118– 119.

4. McAllister, D. R. "Emergency Room Admissions for Drug Related Problems in Los Angeles County Hospitals: A Preliminary Report January-December, 1978." Report No. 80-TA-9, Department of Health Services, Drug Abuse Program Office, Evaluation Unit, Los Angeles, 1980.

5. Strantz, I. H. "The Impact of the PCP Problem on the Los Angeles County Treatment Systems." Paper presented at the PCP Forum, Los Angeles, March 27, 1980.

6. *Microgram* 10(8):98– 101.

7. From discussions at the PCP Conference of the National Institute on Drug Abuse, Asilomar Conference Center, Pacific Grove, California, February 27– 28, 1978.

8. Davies, B. M., and Beech, H. R. "The Effect of 1-Arylcyclohexylamine (Sernyl) on Twelve Normal Volunteers." *Journal of Mental Sciences* 106:912– 924.

9. Domino, E. F. "Neurobiology of Phencyclidine (Sernyl), a Drug with an Unusual Spectrum of Pharmacological Activity." *International Review of Neurobiology* 6:303– 347.

10. Gool, R. V., and Clarke, H. L. "Anaesthesia for Under-Doctored Areas: A Trial of Phencyclidine in Nigeria." *Anaesthesia* 18:265– 270.

11. Pollard, J. C., and Uhr, L. *Drugs and Fantasy: The Effects of LSD, Psilocybin and Sernyl on College Students.* Boston: Little, Brown, 1965, pp. 89– 104 and 131– 136.

12. Ban, J. A.; Lohrenz, J. J.; and Lehmann, H. E. "Observations of the Action of Sernyl — A New Psychotropic Drug." *Canadian Psychiatric Association Journal* 6(3):154.

13. Domino, E. F. "History and Pharmacology of PCP and PCP-Related Analogs." Paper presented at the National Conference on the Problems and Prevention of PCP Abuse, San Francisco, California, November 3, 1979.

14. Waddy, F. F. Letter to the editor. *Anaesthesia* 18(1):117– 119.

15. Gorringe, J. A. L. Letter to the editor. *Anaesthesia* 18(1):117– 119.

16. Authors' interview with chronic phencyclidine user.

17. Burns, R. S., and Lerner, S. E. "Phencyclidine-Related Deaths." *Journal of the American College of Emergency Physicians* 7(4):135– 141.

18. Burns, R. S.; Lerner, S. E.; Corrado, R.; James, S. H.; and Schnoll, S. H. "Phencyclidine — States of Acute Intoxication and Fatalities." *The Western Journal of Medicine* 123(5):345–349.

19. Burns, R. S., and Lerner, S. E. "Street PCP Use: Clinical Studies of the Acute and Chronic Intoxicated State." *Newsletter of the California Association of Toxicologists,* August 1975, pp. 32–59.

20. Lerner, S. E., and Burns, R. S. "Phencyclidine Use Among Youth: History, Epidemiology, and Acute and Chronic Intoxication." In R. C. Peterson and R. C. Stillman, eds., *Phencyclidine Abuse: An Appraisal.* National Institute on Drug Abuse Monograph No. 21, U.S. Department of Health, Education, and Welfare No. (ADM) 78-728. Washington, D.C.: U.S. Government Printing Office, 1978, pp. 66–118.

21. Lundberg, G. D.; Gupta, R. C.; and Montgomery, S. H. "Phencyclidine: Patterns Seen in Street Drug Analysis." *Clinical Toxicology* 9(4):503–511.

22. Perry, D. C. "PCP Revisited." *PharmChem Foundation Newsletter* 4(9):1–7.

23. *Phencyclidine (PCP or Angel Dust),* Joint Hearings before the Subcommittee on Alcoholism and Drug Abuse of the Committee on Human Resources and the Subcommittee to Investigate Juvenile Delinquency of the Committee on the Judiciary, United States Senate, June 7 and 21. Washington, D.C.: U.S. Government Printing Office, 1978.

24. Lerner, S. E., and Linder, R. L. "Phencyclidine Toxicity." *Cathexis* 3(1):22–27.

25. Personal communication with PharmChem Laboratories, Menlo Park, California.

26. Personal communication with U.S. Drug Enforcement Administration, Washington, D.C.

27. Personal communication with Forecasting Branch, National Institute on Drug Abuse, July 29, 1980.

28. Lerner, S. E., and Burns, R. S. "Youthful Phencyclidine (PCP) Users." In G. M. Beschner and A. S. Friedman, eds., *Youth Drug Abuse.* Lexington, Mass.: Lexington Books, 1979, pp. 315–352.

29. "Substance Use Among New York State Public and Parochial School Students in Grades 7 Through 12." New York State Division of Substance Abuse Services, November 1978.

30. Johnston, L. D.; Bachman, J. G.; and O'Malley, P. M. *1979 Highlights, Drugs and the Nation's High School Students.* The University of

**122**

Michigan, Institute for Social Research, U.S. Department of Health, Education, and Welfare Publication No. (ADM) 80-930. Washington, D.C.: U.S. Government Printing Office, 1979.

31. Alcott, H. F. "An Incident Study of PCP Use in an Adult Parole Population." State of California, Department of Corrections, Paroles and Community Services Division, Region III-EMIT Lab, 1979.

32. Testimony on Drugs and the Elderly Presented before the Select Committee on Narcotic Abuse and Control, United States House of Representatives, Ninety-Sixth Congress, June 15, 1978.

33. DuPont, R. L. Letter to drug treatment program directors in the United States, October 30, 1977.

34. Statement by Robert L. DuPont, Director of the National Institute on Drug Abuse, before the American Public Health Association Conference, October 30, 1977.

## Chapter 2

1. Domino, E. F. "Neurobiology of Phencyclidine (Sernyl), a Drug with an Unusual Spectrum of Pharmacological Activity." *International Review of Neurobiology* 6:303– 347.

2. Domino, E. F.; Chodoff, P.; and Corssen, G. "Pharmacologic Effects of CI-581, a New Dissociative Anesthetic in Man." *Clinical Pharmacology and Therapeutics* 6(3):279– 291.

3. Domino, E. F. "Neurobiology of Phencyclidine — An Update." In R. C. Peterson and R. C. Stillman, eds., *Phencyclidine Abuse: An Appraisal.* National Institute on Drug Abuse Monograph No. 21, U.S. Department of Health, Education, and Welfare No. (ADM) 78-728. Washington, D.C.: U.S. Government Printing Office, 1978, pp. 18– 43.

4. Balster, R. L., and Chait, L. C. "The Behavioral Effects of Phencyclidine in Animals." In R. C. Peterson and R. C. Stillman, eds., *Phencyclidine Abuse: An Appraisal.* National Institute on Drug Abuse Monograph No. 21, U.S. Department of Health, Education, and Welfare No. (ADM) 78-728. Washington, D.C.: U.S. Government Printing Office, 1978, pp. 53– 65.

5. Domino, E. F., and Luby, E. D. "Abnormal Mental States Induced by PCP as a Model for Schizophrenia." In J. O. Cole, A. M.

Freedman and A. J. Friedhoff, eds., *Psychopathology and Psychopharmacology.* Baltimore: Johns Hopkins University Press, 1972, pp. 37–50. **123**

6.  Lerner, S. E., and Linder, R. L. *Phencyclidine (PCP) Abuse.* United States Army, 1980.

7.  Burns, R. S., and Lerner, S. E. "The Effects of Phencyclidine in Man: A Review. In E. F. Domino, ed., *PCP (Phencyclidine): Historical and Current Perspectives.* Ann Arbor, Mich.: NPP Books, forthcoming.

8.  James, S. H., and Schnoll, S. H. "Phencyclidine: Tissue Distribution in the Rat." *Clinical Toxicology* 9(4):573–582.

9.  Burns, R. S., and Lerner, S. E. "Perspectives: Acute Phencyclidine Intoxication." *Clinical Toxicology* 9(4):477–501.

10. Burns, R. S.; Lerner, S. E.; Corrado, R.; James, S. H.; and Schnoll, S. H. "Phencyclidine — States of Acute Intoxication and Fatalities." *The Western Journal of Medicine* 123(5):345–349.

11. Lerner, S. E. "Phencyclidine Abuse in the United States." *Proceedings of the Joint Hearings before the Subcommittee on Alcoholism and Drug Abuse of the Committee on Human Resources and the Subcommittee to Investigate Juvenile Delinquency of the Committee on the Judiciary, United States Senate, on Phencyclidine (PCP or Angel Dust).* Washington, D.C.: U.S. Government Printing Office, 1978, pp. 15–22.

12. Lerner, S. E., and Burns, R. S. "Phencyclidine Use Among Youth: History, Epidemiology, and Acute and Chronic Intoxication." In R. C. Peterson and R. C. Stillman, eds., *Phencyclidine Abuse: An Appraisal.* National Institute on Drug Abuse Monograph No. 21, U.S. Department of Health, Education, and Welfare No. (ADM) 78-728. Washington, D.C.: U.S. Government Printing Office, 1978, pp. 66–118.

13. Lerner, S. E., and Burns, R. S. "Youthful Phencyclidine (PCP) Users." In G. M. Beschner and A. S. Friedman, eds., *Youth Drug Abuse.* Lexington, Mass.: Lexington Books, 1979, pp. 315–352.

14. Russ, C., and Wong, D. "Diagnosis and Treatment of the Phencyclidine Psychosis: Clinical Considerations." *Journal of Psychedelic Drugs* 11(4):277–282.

15. Luisada, P. V. "The Phencyclidine Psychosis: Phenomenology and Treatment." In R. C. Peterson and R. C. Stillman, eds., *Phencyclidine Abuse: An Appraisal.* National Institute on Drug Abuse Monograph No. 21, U.S. Department of Health, Education, and Welfare No. (ADM) 78-728. Washington, D.C.: U.S. Government Printing Office, 1978, pp. 241–253.

**124**

16. Luisada, P., and Reddick, C. "An Epidemic of Drug-Induced 'Schizophrenia.'" Paper presented at the 128th annual meeting of the American Psychiatric Association, Anaheim, California, May 5, 1975.

17. Lerner, S. E. "Effects of Chronic Exposure to Phencyclidine on Psychological Functioning." Doctoral dissertation, California School of Professional Psychology at Berkeley, 1979.

18. Lerner, S. E., and Linder, R. L. "Drugs in the Elementary School." *Journal of Drug Education* 4(3):317–322.

19. Linder, R. L.; Lerner, S. E.; and Burke, E. M. "Drugs in the Junior High School, Part I." *Journal of Psychedelic Drugs* 6(1):43–49.

20. Lerner, S. E., and Linder, R. L. "Drugs in the High School." *Journal of Drug Education* 4(2):187–195.

21. *Community and Legal Responses to Drug Paraphernalia.* NIDA Services Research Report, U.S. Department of Health, Education, and Welfare Publication No. (ADM) 80-963. Washington, D.C.: U.S. Government Printing Office, 1980.

22. Personal communication with the Los Angeles Police Department.

23. "The Role of Drugs," *Life and Health,* New York: CRM, Random House, Inc., 1976, p. 81.

24. Fauman, M. A., and Fauman, B. J. "Violence Associated with Phencyclidine Abuse." *American Journal of Psychiatry* 136(12):1584–1586.

25. Simonds, J. F., and Kashani, J. "Phencyclidine Use in Delinquent Males Committed to a Training School." *Adolescence* 14(56):721–725.

26. Newmeyer, J. A. "The Epidemiology of PCP Use in the Late 1970s." Unpublished manuscript.

27. "Clandestine Laboratories," *Orange County Sheriff's Department Training Bulletin,* Volume 3, Bulletin No. 16, 1980.

## Chapter 3

1. Burns, R. S.; Lerner, S. E.; Corrado, R.; James, S. H.; and Schnoll, S. H. "Phencyclidine — States of Acute Intoxication and Fatalities." *The Western Journal of Medicine* 123(5):345–349.

2. Lerner, S. E. "Effects of Chronic Exposure to Phencyclidine on Psychological Functioning." Doctoral dissertation, California School of Professional Psychology at Berkeley, 1979.

3. Burns, R. S., and Lerner, S. E. "The Causes of Phencyclidine-Related Deaths." *Clinical Toxicology* 12(4):527–545.

4. Lerner, S. E. "Phencyclidine Abuse in Perspective." In M. T. McAdams, R. L. Linder, S. E. Lerner, R. S. Burns, eds., *Phencyclidine Abuse Manual*. Los Angeles: University of California Extension, 1980, pp. 12–32.

5. Burns, R. S. "Emergency Medical Management Procedures." In M. T. McAdams, R. L. Linder, S. E. Lerner, R. S. Burns, eds., *Phencyclidine Abuse Manual*. Los Angeles: University of California Extension, 1980, pp. 95–113.

6. Burns, R. S., and Lerner, S. E. "Phencyclidine-Related Deaths." *Journal of the American College of Emergency Physicians* 7(4):135–141.

7. Burns, R. S., and Lerner, S. E. "Street PCP Use: Clinical Studies of Acute and Chronic Intoxicated State." *Newsletter of the California Association of Toxicologists,* August 1975, pp. 32–59.

8. Burns, R. S., and Lerner, S. E. "Perspectives: Acute Phencyclidine Intoxication." *Clinical Toxicology* 9(4):477–501.

9. Burns, R. S., and Lerner, S. E. "Management and Treatment of Acute Phencyclidine Intoxications." In P. E. Bourne, ed., *Acute Drug Abuse Emergencies: A Treatment Manual*. New York: Academic Press, 1976, pp. 297–305.

10. Burns, R. S., and Lerner, S. E. "The Effects of Phencyclidine in Man: A Review." In E. F. Domino, ed., *PCP (Phencyclidine): Historical and Current Perspectives*. Ann Arbor, Mich.: NPP Books, forthcoming.

11. Burns, R. S.; Lerner, S. E.; and Linder, R. L. "The Clinical Picture of Phencyclidine Intoxication." *Current Topics II in Emergency Medicine*. The Medical College of Pennsylvania, forthcoming.

12. Garey, R. E.; Samuels, M. S.; Daul, G. C.; Heath, R. G.; Hite, S. A.; Minyard, F.; and Giblin, V. "Phencyclidine Abuse in New Orleans: Medical, Forensic, and Laboratory Aspects." *Substance and Alcohol Actions/Misuse,* forthcoming.

13. Personal communication with R. E. Garey, April 9, 1980.

14. Done, A. K. "Ion-Trapping in Diagnosis and Treatment." In M. T. McAdams, R. L. Linder, S. E. Lerner, and R. S. Burns, eds., *Phencyclidine Abuse Manual*. Los Angeles: University of California Extension, 1980, pp. 114–120.

15. Domino, E. F. "Comparison of Various Symptoms of Acute Schizophrenia and Those Induced by Phencyclidine." In M. T. McAdams, R. L. Linder, S. E. Lerner, and R. S. Burns, eds., *Phencyclidine Abuse Manual*. Los Angeles: University of California Extension, 1980, p. 159.

**126** Chapter 4

1. Burns, R. S., and Lerner, S. E. "Phencyclidine-Related Deaths." *Journal of the American College of Emergency Physicians* 7(4):135–141.
2. Burns, R. S.; Lerner, S. E.; Corrado, R.; James, S. H.; and Schnoll, S. H. "Phencyclidine — States of Acute Intoxication and Fatalities." *The Western Journal of Medicine* 123(5):345–349.
3. Burns, R. S., and Lerner, S. E. "Perspectives: Acute Phencyclidine Intoxication." *Clinical Toxicology* 9(4):477–501.
4. Burns, R. S., and Lerner, S. E. "Management and Treatment of Acute Phencyclidine Intoxications." In P. E. Bourne, ed., *Acute Drug Abuse Emergencies: A Treatment Manual.* New York: Academic Press, 1976, pp. 297–305.
5. Burns, R. S. "Emergency Medical Management Procedures." In M. T. McAdams, R. L. Linder, S. E. Lerner, R. S. Burns, eds., *Phencyclidine Abuse Manual.* Los Angeles: University of California Extension, 1980, pp. 90–115.
6. Burns, R. S., and Lerner, S. E. "The Effects of Phencyclidine in Man: A Review." In E. F. Domino, ed., *PCP (Phencyclidine): Historical and Current Perspectives.* Ann Arbor, Mich.: NPP Books, forthcoming.
7. Burns, R. S.; Lerner, S. E.; and Linder, R. L. "The Clinical Picture of Phencyclidine Intoxication." *Current Topics II in Emergency Medicine.* The Medical College of Pennsylvania, forthcoming.
8. Eastman, J. W., and Cohen, S. N. "Hypertensive Crisis and Death Associated with Phencyclidine Poisoning." *Journal of the American Medical Association* 231:1270–1271.
9. *A Comparison of Mental Health Treatment Center and Drug Abuse Treatment Center Approaches to Nonopiate Drug Abuse.* National Institute on Drug Abuse Services Research Report, DHEW Publication No. (ADM) 79-879, 1979, p. 13.
10. Luisada, P. V. "Clinical Experience with Phencyclidine Psychosis." In R. C. Peterson and R. C. Stillman, eds., *Phencyclidine Abuse: An Appraisal.* National Institute on Drug Abuse Monograph No. 21, U.S. Department of Health, Education, and Welfare No. (ADM) 78-728.
11. Luisada, P. V., and Reddick, C. "An Epidemic of Drug Induced 'Schizophrenia.'" Paper presented at the 128th annual meeting of the American Psychiatric Association, Anaheim, California, May 5, 1975.

Chapter 5 **127**

1.  Third Annual National Homicide Symposium, San Diego, California, October 22–26, 1979.
2.  Model Penal Code. Article 4, Section 4.01.
3.  Sher, M. D. "Phencyclidine Induced Psychosis and the Insanity Defense." *Criminal Defense* 4(4):5–10.
4.  Fauman, M. A., and Fauman, B. J. "Violence Associated with Phencyclidine Abuse." *American Journal of Psychiatry* 136(12):1586.
5.  Clardy, D., and Ragle, J. L. "Stability of Phencyclidine in Stored Blood." *Clinical Toxicology,* forthcoming.
6.  Burns, R. S.; Lerner, S. E.; Corrado, R.; James, S. H.; and Schnoll, S. H. "Phencyclidine — States of Acute Intoxication and Fatalities." *The Western Journal of Medicine* 123(5):345–349.
7.  Burns, R. S., and Lerner, S. E. "Perspectives: Acute Phencyclidine Intoxication." *Clinical Toxicology* 9(4):477–501.
8.  Burns, R. S., and Lerner, S. E. "Phencyclidine-Related Deaths." *The Journal of the American College of Emergency Physicians* 7(4):135–141.

## 128  Glossary

*Analog:* a related compound with a similar chemical structure

*Aphrodisiac:* enhancement of sexual drive

*Apnea:* stoppage of breathing

*Behavioral toxicity:* inability to appreciate the consequences of one's behavior due to phencyclidine use

*Blank stare:* expressionless face

*Catalepsy:* loss of voluntary motion in which limbs remain in whatever position they are placed

*Cerebral angiograph:* radiograph of vessels supplying blood to the brain

*Cerebral hemorrhage:* bleeding into the brain

*Cerebrovascular accident:* stroke, loss of blood supply to part of the brain with resulting paralysis

*Chronic PCP use:* use of PCP at least three times per week for a period of six months or longer

*Decompensation:* progressive failure of defense mechanisms

*Delta, theta slowing:* low frequency waves representing abnormal brain activity

*Downer:* depressant drugs such as alcohol, opiates, barbiturates

*EEG (Electroencephalogram):* a graphic record of the electrical activity of the brain

*EEG, slow-wave complex:* a series of low frequency waves on the EEG indicating abnormal brain activity

*Endogenous-type depression:* a depressed state produced by internal chemical changes

*Extensor posturing:* rigid extension of limbs

*Focal neurological finding:* a neurological sign indicating focal damage to the brain

*Focal seizure:* a seizure originating in one focus of the brain resulting in abnormal function in one location of the body

*Gait ataxia:* inability to walk heel-to-toe in a straight line

*Generalized seizure:* synchronous abnormal electrical activity throughout the brain resulting in unconsiousness and jerky movements of the limbs

*Hematoma:* a localized collection of blood resulting from a tear in a major vessel

— epidural: a collection of blood between the skull and the thick membrane enclosing the brain
— subdural: a collection of blood between the brain and the thick membrane covering the brain

*Hyperreflexia:* increased tendon jerks

*Hypertension:* high arterial blood pressure

*Hypoventilation:* slowed, shallow breathing

*Ion-trapping effect:* the conversion in gastric fluid or kidney filtrate of a molecule to an ionized form preventing its reabsorption into the body

*Laryngospasm:* abnormal closure of the epiglottis

*Lavage:* flushing out the stomach with water using a nasogastric tube

*Meningitis:* infection of the membrane surrounding the brain or spinal cord

*Microgram:* one millionth of a gram

*Milligram:* one thousandth of a gram

*Milliliter:* one thousandth of a liter

*Myoclonic jerking:* a rapid jerking movement

*Myoglobinuria:* the excretion of myoglobine, a muscle protein, red in color, into the urine

*Nanogram:* one billionth of a gram

*Nasogastric suctioning:* placing a rubber tube from the nose into the stomach and draining the stomach contents

*Nystagmus:* jerky movements of the eyes

*Organic brain syndrome:* changes in higher mental state due to brain dysfunction

*Outer:* hallucinogenic drugs such as LSD, mescaline

*PCP:* 1-(1-phencyclohexyl) piperidine hydrochloride; the prototype drug of the phencyclidines

*PCPer:* an individual who uses the phencyclidines

*Phenytoin* (Dilantin): widely used anticonvulsant

*Phlebitis:* inflammation of a vein

*Polydrug abuse:* abuse of two or more drugs

*Postical state:* coma following a seizure

*Procaine:* a local anesthetic used in medicine and dentistry

*Projective test:* a psychological test in which an individual's personal characteristics are elicited by their response to standardized images

*Psychosis:* inability to differentiate between reality and fantasy

*Psychotomimetic:* a drug that produces psychoses-like symptoms

*Quaalude:* a non-barbiturate sedative

*Schizophrenia:* inability to maintain contact with the real world resulting from personality disintegration

*Tachycardia:* rapid beating of the heart

*Toxic psychosis:* severe impairment of mental functioning caused by a chemical substance

*Upper:* stimulant drugs such as amphetamines, caffeine, nicotine, cocaine

*Wernicke's syndrome or Wernicke's encephalopathy:* organic brain damage caused by vitamin $B^1$ deficiency associated with chronic alcoholism

# Referral Agencies List

### Alabama

Division of Alcoholism and Drug Abuse
Department of Mental Health
135 South Union St.
Montgomery, AL 36130
(205) 265-2301

### Alaska

Department of Health and Social Services
Office of Alcoholism and Drug Abuse
Pouch H-05-F
Juneau, AK 99811
(907) 586-6201 or FTS 8-399-0150

### Arizona

Alcohol Section
Arizona Department of Health Services
2500 East Van Buren
Phoenix, AZ 85008
(602) 271-3009

Drug Abuse Section
Department of Health Services
Division of Behavioral Health Services
2500 East Van Buren
Phoenix, AZ 85008
(602) 255-1239

### Arkansas

Arkansas Office on Alcohol and Drug Abuse Prevention
1515 W. 7th Avenue, Suite 300
Little Rock, AR 72205
(501) 371-2604

### California

Department of Alcohol and Drug Programs
111 Capital Mall
Sacramento, CA 95814
(916) 445-1940 or 322-8484

### Colorado

Alcohol and Drug Abuse Division
Department of Health
4210 East 11th Avenue
Denver, CO 80220
(303) 320-8333

### Connecticut

Connecticut Alcohol and Drug Abuse Council
90 Washington Street, Room 312
Hartford, CT 06115
(203) 566-4145

### Delaware

Bureau of Substance Abuse
1901 N. Dupont Highway
Newcastle, DE 19720
(302) 421-6101

### District of Columbia

Mental Health, Alcohol and Addiction Services Branch
1329 E Street, N.W.
Suite 1034
Washington, DC 20004
(202) 724-5641

Florida

Alcoholic Rehabilitation Program
Department of Health and
Rehabilitation Services
1323 Winewood Boulevard
Tallahassee, FL 32301
(904) 487-2820

Drug Abuse Program
1309 Winewood Boulevard
Building 6
Tallahassee, FL 32301
(904) 488-0900

Georgia

Alcohol and Drug Section
Division of Mental Health and
Mental Retardation
Georgia Department of Human
Resources
618 Ponce de Leon Avenue, N.E.
Atlanta, GA 30308
(404) 894-4785

Hawaii

Alcohol and Drug Abuse Branch
1270 Queen Emma Street, Room
404
Honolulu, HI 96813
(808) 548-7655

Idaho

Bureau of Substance Abuse
Department of Health and Welfare
700 West State
Boise, ID 83720
(208) 384-7706

Illinois

Alcohol Division
Illinois Department of Mental

Health and Developmental Disabilities
160 North LaSalle Street,
Room 1500
Chicago, IL 60601
(312) 793-2907

Illinois Dangerous Drugs
Commission
300 North State Street
Suite 1500
Chicago, IL 60610
(312) 822-9860

Indiana

Division of Addiction Services
Department of Mental Health
5 Indiana Square
Indianapolis, IN 46204
(317) 633-4477

Iowa

Department of Substance Abuse
Liberty Building, Suite 230
418 Sixth Avenue
Des Moines, IA 50319
(515) 281-3641

Kansas

Alcoholism and Drug Abuse
Section
2700 West Sixth Street
Biddle Building
Topeka, KS 66606
(913) 296-3925

Kentucky

Alcohol and Drug Branch
Bureau of Health Services
Department of Human Resources
275 East Main Street
Frankfort, KY 40621
(502) 564-7450

## Louisiana

Bureau of Substance Abuse
Department of Health and Human
Resources
200 Lafayette Street
Baton Rouge, LA 70801
(504) 342-2575

## Maine

Office of Alcoholism and Drug
Abuse Prevention
Bureau of Rehabilitation
32 Winthrop Street
Augusta, ME 04330
(207) 289-2781

## Maryland

Alcoholism Control
Administration
201 West Preston Street, 4th Floor
Baltimore, MD 21201
(301) 383-2781, 2782, 2783

Maryland State Drug Abuse
Administration
201 West Preston Street
Baltimore, MD 21201
(301) 383-7404

## Massachusetts

Massachusetts Division of
Alcoholism
755 Boylston Street
Boston, MA 02116
(617) 727-1960

Division of Drug Rehabilitation
160 N. Washington Street
Boston, MA 02114
(617) 727-8614

## Michigan

Office of Substance Abuse
Services
Department of Public Health
3500 North Logan Street
Lansing, MI 48914
(517) 373-8600

## Minnesota

Chemical Dependency Program
Division
Department of Public Welfare
4th Floor Centennial Building
658 Cedar
St. Paul, MN 55155
(612) 296-4610

## Mississippi

Division of Alcohol and Drug
Abuse
Department of Mental Health
619 Robert E. Lee State Office
Building
Jackson, MS 32901
(601) 354-7031

## Missouri

Division of Alcoholism and Drug
Abuse
Department of Mental Health
2002 Missouri Boulevard
P.O. Box 687
Jefferson City, MO 65101
(314) 751-4942

## Montana

Alcohol and Drug Abuse Division
State of Montana
Department of Institutions
Helena, MT 59601
(406) 449-2827

### Nebraska

Nebraska Division of Alcoholism
Box 94728
Lincoln, NB 68509
(402) 471-2851

Nebraska Commission on Drugs
P.O. Box 94726
Nebraska State Office Building
Lincoln, NB 68509
(402) 471-2691

### Nevada

Bureau of Alcohol and Drug
Abuse
Department of Human Resources
505 East King Street
Carson City, NV 89710
(702) 885-4790

### New Hampshire

New Hampshire Program on
Alcohol and Drug Abuse
61 South Spring Street
Concord, NH 03301
(603) 271-3531

Office of Substance Abuse
Office of the Governor
3 Capitol Street, 405
Concord, NH 03301
(603) 271-2754

### New Jersey

New Jersey Division of
Alcoholism
129 East Hanover Street
Trenton, NJ 08625
(609) 292-8947

Division of Narcotic and
Drug Abuse Control
129 East Hanover Street
Trenton, NJ 08625
(609) 292-5760

### New Mexico

Substance Abuse Bureau
Behavioral Services Division
Health and Environment
Department
P.O. Box 968
Santa Fe, NM 87503
(505) 827-5271 Ext. 228

### New York

New York Division of
Alcoholism and Alcohol Abuse
44 Holland Avenue
Albany, NY 12208
(518) 474-5417

Division of Substance Abuse
Services
Executive Park South, Box 8200
Albany, NY 12203
(518) 457-7629

### North Carolina

Alcohol and Drug Abuse Section
Division of Mental Health and
Mental Retardation Services
325 North Salisbury Street
Raleigh, NC 27611
(919) 733-4670

Alcohol and Drug Abuse Section
Department of Human Resources
325 North Salisbury Street
Raleigh, NC 27611
(919) 733-6650

## North Dakota

Division of Alcoholism and Drug Abuse
Mental Health/Mental Retardation Services
State Department of Health
909 Basin Avenue
Bismarck, ND 58505
(701) 224-2767

## Ohio

Division of Alcoholism
Ohio Department of Health
246 North High Street
Columbus, OH 43215
(614) 466-3425

Bureau of Drug Abuse
65 South Front Street
Suite 211
Columbus, OH 43215
(614) 466-9023

## Oklahoma

State Alcohol Authority
P.O. Box 53277, Capitol Station
Oklahoma City, OK 73152
(405) 521-2811

Drug Abuse Services
State Department of Mental Health
P.O. Box 53277, Capitol Station
Oklahoma City, OK 73152
(405) 521-2811

## Oregon

Program for Alcohol and Drug Problems
Oregon Mental Health Division

2575 Bittern Street, N.E.
Salem, OR 97310
(503) 378-2163

Drug Abuse Program
Mental Health Division
2575 Bittern Street, N.E.
Salem, OR 97310
(503) 378-2163

## Pennsylvania

Governor's Council on Drug and Alcohol Abuse
Riverside Office, Bldg. #1, Suite N
2101 North Front Street
Harrisburg, PA 17120
(717) 787-9857

## Rhode Island

Division of Substance Abuse
303 General Hospital
Rhode Island Medical Center
Cranston, RI 02920
(401) 464-2091

## South Carolina

South Carolina Commission on Alcohol and Drug Abuse
3700 Forest Drive
Columbia, SC 29204
(803) 758-2521/2183

## South Dakota

South Dakota Division of Alcoholism
Joe Foss Building
Pierre, SD 57501
(605) 773-4806

**135**

**136**

Division of Drugs and Substance
Control
Department of Health
Joe Foss Building
Pierre, SD 57501
(605) 773-3123

### Tennessee

Alcohol and Drug Abuse Services
Tennessee Department of Mental
Health and Mental Retardation
501 Union Building
Nashville, TN 37219
(615) 741-1921

### Texas

Texas Commission on Alcoholism
809 Sam Houston State Office
Building
Austin, TX 78701
(512) 475-2725

Drug Abuse Prevention Division
Texas Department of Community
Affairs
P.O. Box 13166
Austin, TX 78711
(512) 475-6351

### Utah

Division of Alcoholism and Drugs
150 West North Temple, Suite 350
P.O. Box 2500
Salt Lake City, UT 84110
(801) 533-6532

### Vermont

Alcohol and Drug Abuse Division
Department of Social and
Rehabilitation Services

State Office Building
Montpelier, VT 05602
(802) 241-2170, 241-1000

### Virginia

Division of Substance Abuse
State Department of Mental
Health and Mental Retardation
P.O. Box 1797
109 Governor Street
Richmond, VA 23214
(804) 786-5313

### Washington

Bureau of Alcoholism and
Substance Abuse
Washington Department of Social
and Health Services Office
Building
Olympia, WA 98504
(206) 753-3073

### West Virginia

Division of Alcohol and Drug
Abuse
State Capitol
1800 Kanawha Boulevard E
Charleston, WV 25305
(304) 348-3616

### Wisconsin

State Bureau of Alcohol and
Other Drug Abuse
One West Wilson Street,
Room 523
Madison, WI 53702
(608) 266-2717

Wyoming

Alcohol and Alcohol Abuse
Programs
Hathaway Building
Cheyenne, WY 82002
(307) 777-7115 Ext. 7118

Puerto Rico

Puerto Rico Department of
Addiction Control Services
Box B-Y, Rio Piedras Station
Rio Piedras, PR 00928
(809) 763-5014 or 7575

Department of Addiction Control
Services
P.O. Box B-Y
Piedras Station, PR 00928
(809) 764-8140

American Samoa

Mental Health Clinic
Government of American Samoa
Pago Pago, AS 96799

Guam

Mental Health and Substance
Abuse Agency
Single State Agency
P.O. Box 20999
Guam, GU 96921

Virgin Islands

Division of Mental Health,
Alcoholism and Drug
Dependency
P.O. Box 520
Christiansted
St. Croix, VI 00820
(809) 774-4888 Dial Direct, or
(809) 249-7959

Trust Territories

Health Services
Office of the High Commissioner
Saipan, TT 96950
FTS 8-556-0220, 9422 or 9355

For Technical Information

National Institute on Drug Abuse
National Clearinghouse for Drug
Abuse Information
5600 Fishers Lane
Room 10A56
Rockville, MD 20857

Drs. Lerner, Burns, Linder and
Associates
350 Parnassus Avenue
Suite 304-A
San Francisco, CA 94117
(415) 752-9269

# 138 Bibliography

Abram, M.; Tagger, M.; and Perlmutter, S. "Phencyclidine-Induced Anesthesia for Dental Procedures in the Baboon." *Journal of Dental Research* 52:630.

Alan, R. M., and Young, S. J. "Phencyclidine-Induced Psychosis." *American Journal of Psychiatry* 135:1081 – 1084.

Aronow, R., and Done, A. K. "Phencyclidine Overdose: Emerging Concepts of Treatment." *Journal of the American College of Emergency Physicians* 7(2): 56 – 59.

Aronow, R.; Miceli, J. N.; and Done, A. K. "Clinical Observations during Phencyclidine Intoxication and Treatment Based on Ion-Trapping." In R. C. Peterson and R. C. Stillman, eds., *Phencyclidine Abuse: An Appraisal*. NIDA Monograph No. 21, U.S. Department of Health, Education, and Welfare No. (ADM) 78-728. Washington, D.C.: U.S. Government Printing Office, 1978.

Bakker, C. B., and Amini, F. B. "Observations on the Psychotomimetic Effects of Sernyl." *Comprehensive Psychiatry* 2:269 – 280.

Balkrishena, K., and Davidow, B. "Radioimmunoassay Screening for Detection of Phencyclidine (PCP, "Angel Dust") Abuse among Teenagers." *Clinical Toxicology* 16(1):7 – 15.

Balster, R. L., and Chait, L. D. "The Behavioral Effects of Phencyclidine in Animals." In R. C. Peterson and R. C. Stillman, eds., *Phencyclidine Abuse: An Appraisal*. NIDA Monograph No. 21, U.S. Department of Health, Education, and Welfare No. (ADM) 78-728. Washington, D.C.: U.S. Government Printing Office, 1978.

Balster, R. L.; Johanson, C. E.; Harris, R. T.; and Schuster, C. R. "Phencyclidine Self-Administration in the Rhesus Monkey." *Pharmacology, Biochemistry, and Behavior* 1:167 – 172.

Balster, R. L., and Woolverton, W. L. "Intravenous Phencyclidine Self-Administration by Rhesus Monkeys Leading to Physical Dependence." In Louis S. Harris, ed., *Problems of Drug Depen-*

*dence 1979,* Proceedings of the 41st Annual Scientific Meeting, **139** The Committee on Problems of Drug Dependence, Inc. NIDA Monograph No. 27, U.S. Department of Health, Education, and Welfare No. (ADM) 80-901. Washington, D.C.: U.S. Government Printing Office, 1980.

Ban, T. A.; Lohrenz, J. J.; and Lehmann, H. E. "Observations on the Action of Sernyl — A New Psychotropic Drug. *Canadian Psychiatric Association Journal* 6:150–156.

Baselt, R. C.; Casarett, L. J.; and Winn, N. E. "Illicit Drugs: Chemical Identity Versus Alleged Identity." *Drug Forum* 1:263–267.

Baselt, R. C.; Wright, J. A.; and Cravey, R. II. "Therapeutic and Toxic Concentrations of More than 100 Toxicologically Significant Drugs in Blood, Plasma, or Serum: A Tabulation." *Clinical Chemistry* 21:44–62.

Beech, H. R.; Davics, B. M.; and Morgenstern, F. S. "Preliminary Investigations of the Effects of Sernyl upon Cognitive and Sensory Processes." *Journal of Mental Science* 107:509–513.

Bodi, T.; Share, I.; Levy, H.; and Moyer, J. H. "Clinical Trial of Phencyclidine (Sernyl) in Patients with Psychoneurosis." *Antibiotic Medicine and Clinical Therapy* 6:79–84.

Bolter, A.; Hemminger, A.; Martin, G.; and Fry, M. "Out-Patient Clinical Experience in a Community Drug Abuse Program with Phencyclidine Abuse." *Clinical Toxicology* 9(4):593–600.

Burns, R. S. "Emergency Medical Management Procedures." In M. T. McAdams, R. L. Linder, S. E. Lerner, and R. S. Burns, eds., *Phencyclidine Abuse Manual.* Los Angeles: University of California Extension, 1980.

Burns, R. S., and Lerner, S. E. "The Causes of Phencyclidine-Related Deaths." *Clinical Toxicology,* 12(4):527–545.

Burns, R. S., and Lerner, S. E. "The Effects of Phencyclidine in Man: A Review." In E. F. Domino, ed., *PCP (Phencyclidine): Historical and Current Perspectives.* Ann Arbor, Mich.: NPP Books, forthcoming.

Burns, R. S., and Lerner, S. E. "Management and Treatment of Acute Phencyclidine Intoxications." In P. E. Bourne, ed., *Acute*

**140**

*Drug Abuse Emergencies: A Treatment Manual.* New York: Academic Press, 1976, pp. 297–305.

Burns, R. S., and Lerner, S. E. "Perspectives: Acute Phencyclidine Intoxication." *Clinical Toxicology* 9(4):477–501.

Burns, R. S., and Lerner, S. E. "Perspectives: Acute Phencyclidine Intoxication (revised)." *Proceedings of the 38th Annual Scientific Meeting, Committee on Problems of Drug Dependence, National Academy of Sciences.* Richmond, Virginia: 1976, pp. 552–574.

Burns, R. S., and Lerner, S. E. "The Phencyclidine Dilemma." *Newsletter of the California Society for the Treatment of Alcoholism and Other Drug Dependencies* 3(2):1–3.

Burns, R. S., and Lerner, S. E. "Phencyclidine: An Emerging Drug Problem." *Clinical Toxicology* 9(4):473–475.

Burns, R. S., and Lerner, S. E. "Phencyclidine-Related Deaths." *Journal of the American College of Emergency Physicians* 7(4):135–141.

Burns, R. S., and Lerner, S. E. "Street PCP Use: Clinical Studies of the Acute and Chronic Intoxicated State." *Newsletter of the California Association of Toxicologists,* August 1975, pp. 32–59.

Burns, R. S.; Lerner, S. E.; Corrado, R.; James, S. H.; and Schnoll, S. H. "Phencyclidine — States of Acute Intoxication and Fatalities." *The Western Journal of Medicine* 123(5):345–349.

Burns, R. S.; Lerner, S. E.; and Linder, R. L. "The Clinical Picture of Phencyclidine Intoxication." *Current Topics II in Emergency Medicine,* The Medical College of Pennsylvania, forthcoming.

Camilleri, J. G. "The Use of Phencyclidine (CI-395) in Obstetric Procedures." *Anaesthesia* 17:422–426.

Camilleri, J. G. "The Use of Phencyclidine (CI-395) for Premedication of Children. *Anaesthesia* 17:419–421.

Catenacci, A. J.; Grove, D. D.; Weiss, W. A.; Fisher, S. M.; Sismondo, A. M.; and Moyer, J. H. "Evaluation of Phencyclidine as a Preanesthetic and Anesthetic Agent." *Antibiotic Medicine and Clinical Therapy* 6:145–150.

Chait, L. D., and Balster, R. L. "The Effects of Acute and Chronic Phencyclidine on Schedule-Controlled Behavior in the Squirrel

Monkey." *The Journal of Pharmacology and Experimental Therapeutics* 204:77–87.

**141**

Chen, G. "Sympathomimetic Anesthetics." *Canadian Anaesthetists Society Journal* 20(2):335–342.

Chen, G.; Ensor, C. R.; and Bohner, B. "An Investigation on the Sympathomimetic Properties of Phencyclidine by Comparison with Cocaine and Desoxyephedrine." *The Journal of Pharmacology and Experimental Therapeutics* 149:71–78.

Chen, G.; Ensor, C. R.; and Bohner, B. "The Neuropharmacology of 2-(0-Chlorohphy)-2-methylamino-cyclohexanone Hydrochloride." *The Journal of Pharmacology and Experimental Therapeutics* 152:332–342.

Chen, G.; Ensor, C. R.; Russell, D.; and Bohner, B. "The Pharmacology of 1-(1-Phenylcyclohexyl)piperidine • HCL." *Journal of Pharmacology and Experimental Therapeutics* 127:241–250.

Chen, G. M., and Weston, J. K. "The Analgesic and Anesthetic Effect of 1-(1-Phenylcyclohexyl) piperidine • HCL on the Monkey." *Anesthesia and Analgesia, Current Researches* 39:132–137.

Chen, G.; Weston, K.; and Weston, J. K. "The Neuropharmacology and Toxicity of Phenylcyclohexylpiperidine HCL." In P. B. Gradley, P. Deniker, and C. Radouco-Thomas, eds., *Neuropsychopharmacology*. Volume 1. Amsterdam: Elsevier, 1959, pp. 294–295.

Clardy, D., and Ragle, J. L. "Stability of Phencyclidine in Stored Blood." *Clinical Toxicology,* forthcoming.

Cohen, B. D.; Rosenbaum, G.; Luby, E. D.; and Gottlieb, J. S. "Comparison of Phencyclidine Hydrochloride (Sernyl) with Other Drugs." *Archives of General Psychiatry* 6:395–401.

Cohen, B. D.; Rosenbaum, G.; Luby, E. D.; and Gottlieb, J. S. "Comparison of Phencyclidine Hydrochloride (Sernyl) with Other Drugs." *Archives of General Psychiatry* 6:79–85.

Cohen, B. D.; Luby, E. D.; Rosenbaum, G.; and Gottlieb, J. S. "Combined Sernyl and Sensory Deprivation." *Comprehensive Psychiatry* 1:345–348.

Cohen, S. "Angel Dust." *Journal of the American Medical Association* 238:515–516.

**142**

Collins, V. J.; Gorospe, C. A.; and Rovenstine, E. A. "Intravenous Nonbarbiturate, Nonnarcotic Analgesics: Preliminary Studies. 1. Cyclohexylamines." *Anesthesia and Analgesia, Current Researches* 39:302– 306.

Corssen, G., and Domino, E. F. "Dissociative Anesthesia: Further Pharmacologic Studies and First Clinical Experience with the Phencyclidine Derivative CI-581." *Anesthesia and Analgesia, Current Researches* 45:29– 40.

Corssen, G.; Miyasaka, M.; and Domino, E. F. "Changing Concepts in Pain Control During Surgery. Dissociative Anesthesia with CI-581, A Progress Report." *Anesthesia and Analgesia, Current Researches* 474:746– 749.

Davies, B. M. "Oral Sernyl in Obsessive States." *Journal of Mental Science* 107:109– 114.

Davies, B. M. "Phencyclidine: Its Use in Psychiatry." In R. Crocket, R. A. Sandison, and A. S. Walk, eds., *Hallucinogenic Drugs and Their Psychotherapeutic Use.* London: H. K. Lewis, 1963, pp. 42– 47.

Davies, B. M. "A Preliminary Report on the Use of Sernyl in Psychiatric Illness." *Journal of Mental Science* 106:1073– 1079.

Davies, B. M., and Beech, H. R. "The Effect of 1-Arylcyclohexylamine (Sernyl) on Twelve Normal Volunteers." *Journal of Mental Sciences* 106:912– 924.

Domino, E. F. "Comparison of Various Symptoms of Acute Schizophrenia and Those Induced by Phencyclidine." In M. T. McAdams, R. L. Linder, S. E. Lerner, R. S. Burns, eds., *Phencyclidine Abuse Manual.* Los Angeles: University of California Extension, 1980, p. 159.

Domino, E. F. "Neurobiology of Phencyclidine (Sernyl), a Drug with an Unusual Spectrum of Pharmacological Activity." *International Review of Neurobiology* 6:303– 347.

Domino, E. F. "Neurobiology of Phencyclidine — An Update." In R. C. Peterson and R. C. Stillman, eds., *Phencyclidine Abuse: An Appraisal.* NIDA Monograph No. 21, U.S. Department of Health, Education, and Welfare No. (ADM) 78-728. Washington, D.C.: U.S. Government Printing Office, 1978.

Domino, E. F. "Some Aspects of the Pharmacology of Phency-  **143** clidine." From *Technical Review of the Psychopharmacology of Hallucinogens*. Sponsored by the National Institute of Drug Abuse, October 21–22, 1976, Bethesda, Md. Published 1978.

Domino, E. F. "Treatment of Phencyclidine Intoxication." *Journal of the American Medical Association* 241(23):2505–2506.

Domino, E. F.; Chodoff, P.; and Corssen, G. "Pharmacologic Effects of CI-581, a New Dissociative Anesthetic in Man." *Clinical Pharmacology and Therapeutics* 6(3):279–291.

Domino, E. F., and Luby, E. D. "Abnormal Mental States Induced by PCP as a Model for Schizophrenia." In J. O. Cole, A. M. Freedman, and A. J. Friedhoff, eds., *Psychopathology and Psychopharmacology*. Baltimore: Johns Hopkins University Press, 1972, pp. 37–50.

Domino, E. F., and Wilson, A. E. "Effects of Urine Acidification on Plasma and Urine Phencyclidine Levels in Overdosage." *Clinical Pharmacology and Therapeutics* 22:421–424.

Donaldson, R. O., and Baselt, R. C. "CSF Phencyclidine." *American Journal of Psychiatry* 136(10):1341–1342.

Done, A. K. "The Toxic Emergency: A Phencyclidine Pin-up." *Emergency Medicine* 10(5):179–182.

Done, A. K.: Aronow, R.; and Micheli, J. N. "Pharmacokinetics of Phencyclidine (PCP) Overdose and Its Treatment." In R. C. Peterson and R. C. Stillman, eds., *Phencyclidine Abuse: An Appraisal*. NIDA Monograph No. 21, U.S. Department of Health, Education, and Welfare No. (ADM) 78-728. Washington, D.C.: U.S. Government Printing Office, 1978.

Done, A. K.; Aronow, R.; Miceli, J.; and Cohen, S. "Pharmacokinetic Bases for the Treatment of Phencyclidine (PCP) Intoxication." *Veterinary and Human Toxicology* 21:104.

Done, A. K.; Aronow, R.; Miceli, J. N.; and Lin, D. C. "Pharmacokinetic Observations in the Treatment of Phencyclidine Poisoning. A Preliminary Report." In B. H. Rumack and A. R. Temple, eds., *Management of the Poisoned Patient*. Princeton: Science Press, 1977, pp. 79–102.

**144**

Eastman, J. W., and Cohen, S. N. "Hypertensive Crisis and Death Associated with Phencyclidine Poisoning." *Journal of the American Medical Association* 231:1270–1271.

Fauman, B.; Aldinger, G.; Fauman, M.; and Rosen, P. "Psychiatric Sequellae of Phencyclidine Abuse." *Clinical Toxicology* 9(4):529–538.

Fauman, B.; Baker, F.; Coppleson, L. W.; Rosen, P.; and Segal, M. B. "Psychosis Induced by Phencyclidine." *Journal of the American College of Emergency Physicians* 4(3):223–225.

Fauman, M. A., and Fauman, B. J. "The Differential Diagnosis of Organic Based Psychiatric Disturbance in the Emergency Department." *Journal of the American College of Emergency Physicians* 6(7):315–323.

Fauman, M. A., and Fauman, B. J. "The Psychiatric Aspect of Chronic Phencyclidine (PCP) Use, a Study of Chronic Phencyclidine Users." In R. C. Peterson and R. C. Stillman, eds., *Phencyclidine Abuse: An Appraisal*. NIDA Monograph No. 21, U.S. Department of Health, Education, and Welfare No. (ADM) 78-728. Washington, D.C.: U.S. Government Printing Office, 1978.

Fauman, M. A., and Fauman, B. J. "Violence Associated with Phencyclidine Abuse." *American Journal of Psychiatry* 136(12):1584–1586, December, 1979.

Finnegan, K. T.; Kanner, M. I.; and Meltzer, H. Y. "Phencyclidine-Induced Rotational Behavior in Rats with Nigrostrial Lesions and Its Modulation by Dopaminergic and Cholinergic Agents." *Pharmacology, Biochemistry, and Behavior* 5:651–660.

Garey, R. E., and Heath, R. G. "The Effects of Phencyclidine on the Uptake of ³H-Catecholamines by Rat Striatal and Hypothalmic Synaptosomes." *Life Sciences* 18:1105–1110.

Garey, R. E.; McQuitty, S.; Tootle, D.; and Heath, R. G. "The Effects of Apomorphine and Haldol on PCP Induced Behavioral and Motor Abnormalities in the Rat." *Life Sciences* 26(4):277–284.

Garey, R. E.; Samuels, M. S.; Daul, G. C.; Heath, R. G.; Hite, S. A.; Minyard, F.; and Giblin, V. "Phencyclidine Abuse in New

Orleans: Medical, Forensic, and Laboratory Effects." *Substance and Alcohol Action/Misuse,* forthcoming.

Garey, R. E.; Wiseberg, L. A.; and Heath, R. G. "Phencyclidine: An Overview." *Journal of Psychedelic Drugs* 9(4):280–285.

Gershon, S., and Olariu, J. "JB 329 — A New Psychotomimetic. Its Antagonism by Tetrahydroaminacrin and Its Comparison with LSD, Mescaline, and Sernyl." *Journal of Neuropsychiatry* 1:377–380.

Golden, N. L.; Sokol, R. J.; and Rubin, I. L. "Angel Dust: Possible Effects on the Fetus." *Pediatrics* 65(1):18–20.

Gool, R. Y., and Clarke, H. L. "Anesthesia for Under-Doctored Areas: A Trial of Phencyclidine in Nigeria." *Anaesthesia* 18:265–270.

Greifenstein, F. E.; Yoshitake, J.; DeVault, M.; and Gejewski, J. E. "A Study of a 1-Aryl cyclo hexyl amine for Anesthesia." *Anesthesia and Analgesia, Current Researches* 37:283–294.

Grove, V. E. "Painless Self-Injury After Ingestion of 'Angel Dust.'" *Journal of the American Medical Association* 242(7):655.

Grove, V. E., Jr. "Phencyclidine (Angel Dust) Invades Texas." *Texas Medicine* 75(5):64–65.

Gupta, R. C.; Lu, I.; Oei, G. L.; and Lundberg, G. D. "Analysis of Phencyclidine (PCP) in Illicit Street Samples and Urine." *Clinical Toxicology* 8(6):611.

Helisten, C., and Shulgin, A. T. "The Detection of 1-Piperidine cyclohexanecarbonitrile (PCC) Contamination in Illicit Preparation of PCP (1-(1-Phenylcyclo-hexyl)-piperidine) and TCP (1-(1-(2-Thienyl)-cyclohexyl)-piperidine)." *Journal of Chromatography* 117:232–240.

Helrich, M., and Atwood, J. M. "Modification of Sernyl Anesthesia with Haloperidol." *Anesthesia and Analgesia, Current Researches* 43:471–474.

Hinko, P. J.; Wendt, W.; Wollin, L. R.; and Massopust, L. C. "Neurophysiologic and Behavioral Effects of Certain Anesthetics Administered Intramuscularly in the Rhesus Monkey *(Macaca Mulatta)*." *American Journal of Veterinary Research* 31:1661–1678.

**146**

Hitner, H., and Di Gregorio, J. "Preliminary Investigation of the Peripheral Sympathomimetic Effects of Phencyclidine." *Archives Internationales de Pharmacodynamine et Therapie* 212:36–42.

Hitzeman, R. J.; Loh, H. H.; and Domino, E. F. "Effect of Phencyclidine on the Accumulation of $^{14}$C-catecholamines Formed from $^{14}$C-tyrosine." *Archives Internationales de Pharmacodynamine et Therapie* 202:252–258.

Hott, L. R. "Angel Dust." *American Journal of Psychiatry* 131:1411.

Ilett, K. F.; Jarrott, B.; O'Donnell, S. R.; and Wanstall, J. C. "Mechanism of Cardiovascular Actions of 1-(1-Phencyclohexyl) piperidine hydrochloride (phencyclidine)." *British Journal of Pharmacology* 28:73–83.

Itil, T.; Keskiner, A.; Kiremitci, N.; and Holden, J. M. "Effect of Phencyclidine in Chronic Schizophrenics." *Canadian Psychiatric Association Journal* 12:209–212.

James, S. H.; Calendrillo, B.; and Schnoll, S. H. "Medical and Toxicological Aspects of the Watkins Glen Rock Concert." Paper presented at the 26th Annual Meeting of the American Academy of Forensic Sciences, Dallas, February 1974.

James, S. H., and Schnoll, S. H. "Phencyclidine: Tissue Distribution in the Rat." *Clinical Toxicology* 9(4):573–582.

Jarbe, T. U. C.; Johansson, J. O.; and Henricksson, B. G. "Drug Discrimination in Rats: The Effects of Phencyclidine and Ditran." *Psychopharmacologia* 42:33–39.

Jasinski, D. R.; Cone, E. J.; Gorodetsky, C. W.; Risner, M. E.; Shannon, H. E.; Su, T. P.; and Vaupel, D. B. "Progress Report from the NIDA Addiction Research Center." In Louis S. Harris, ed., *Problems of Drug Dependence 1979,* Proceedings of the 41st Annual Scientific Meeting, The Committee on Problems of Drug Dependence, Inc., NIDA Monograph No. 27, U.S. Department of Health, Education, and Welfare No. (ADM) 80-901. Washington, D.C.: U.S. Government Printing Office, 1980.

Joffe, M. H. "An Anesthetic for the Chimpanzee; 1-(1-Phenylcyclohexyl) piperidine · HCL." *Anesthesia and Analgesia,*

Johnson, K. M. "Neurochemical Pharmacology of Phency-

clidine." In R. C. Peterson and R. C. Stillman, eds., *Phencyclidine* **147**
*Abuse: An Appraisal.* NIDA Monograph No. 21, U.S. Department of Health, Education, and Welfare No. (ADM) 78-728. Washington, D.C.: U.S. Government Printing Office, 1978.

Johnstone, M. "The Use of Sernyl in Clinical Anesthesia." *Der Anestheist* 9:114–115, 1960.

Johnstone, M.; Evans, V.; and Baigel, S. "Sernyl (CI-395) in Clinical Anaesthesia." *British Journal of Anaesthesia* 31:433–439.

Kanner, M.; Finnegan, K.; and Meltzer, H. Y. "Dopaminergic Effects of Phencyclidine in Rats with Nigrostriatal Lesions." *Psychopharmacology Communications* 1(4):393–401.

Kessler, G. F.; Demers, L. M.; Berlin, C.; and Brennan, R. W. "Phencyclidine and Fatal Status Epilepticus." *New England Journal of Medicine* 291:979.

Kuroda, T., and McNamara, J. A. "The Effect of Ketamine and Phencyclidine on Muscle Activity in Nonhuman Primates." *Anesthesia and Analgesia, Current Researches* 51:710–716.

Kurtzke, J. F. "The Use of Cyclohexylamines in Thalamic Pain." *Neurology* 11(5):390–394.

Lambert, C. "The Value of Intravenous Phencyclidine (Sernyl) in the Treatment of Neurosis." In P. B. Bradley, F. Flugel, and P. H. Hoch, eds., *Neuropsychopharmacology. 3.* Amsterdam: Elsevier, 1964, pp. 365–369.

Lawes, T. G. "Schizophrenia, 'Sernyl' and Sensory Deprivation." *British Journal of Psychiatry* 109:243–250.

Lees, H. "The Effect in Vitro of 1-(1-Phenylcyclohexyl) piperidine hydrochloride (Sernyl) on Respiratory and Related Reactions of Liver Mitochondria in Vitro." *Biochemical Pharmacology* 17:845–848.

Leonard, B. E., and Tonge, S. R. "Some Biochemical and Pharmacological Properties of Phencyclidine." *British Journal of Pharmacology and Chemotherapy* 32:415–416, 1968.

Leonard, B. E., and Tonge, S. R. "Some Effects of an Hallucinogenic Drug (Phencyclidine) on Neurohumoral Substances." *Life Sciences* 9:1141–1152.

**148**

Lerner, S. E. "The Effects of Chronic Exposure to Phencyclidine on Psychological Functioning." Doctoral Dissertation, California School of Professional Psychology at Berkeley, 1979.

Lerner, S. E. "Phencyclidine Abuse in Perspective." In M. T. McAdams, R. L. Linder, S. E. Lerner, and R. S. Burns, eds., *Phencyclidine Abuse Manual.* Los Angeles: University of California Extension, 1980, pp. 13–23.

Lerner, S. E. "Phencyclidine Abuse in the United States." In *Proceedings of the Joint Hearings before the Subcommittee on Alcoholism and Drug Abuse of the Committee on Human Resources and the Subcommittee to Investigate Juvenile Delinquency of the Committee on the Judiciary, United States Senate on Phencyclidine (PCP or Angel Dust).* Washington, D.C.: U.S. Government Printing Office, 1978.

Lerner, S. E., and Burns, R. S. "Phencyclidine Use Among Youth; History, Epidemiology, and Acute and Chronic Intoxication." In R. C. Peterson and R. C. Stillman, eds., *Phencyclidine Abuse: An Appraisal.* NIDA Monograph No. 21, U.S. Department of Health, Education, and Welfare No. (ADM) 78-728. Washington, D.C.: U.S. Government Printing Office, 1978.

Lerner, S. E., and Burns, R. S. "Youthful Phencyclidine (PCP) Users." In G. M. Beschener and A. S. Friedman, eds., *Youth Drug Abuse.* Lexington, Mass.: Lexington Books, 1979.

Lerner, S. E., and Linder, R. L. *Phencyclidine (PCP) Abuse.* Department of Defense, 1980.

Lerner, S. E., and Linder, R. L. "Phencyclidine Toxicity." *Cathexis* 3(1):22–27.

Levy, L.; Cameron, E. D.; and Aitken, C. B. "Observation on Two Psychotomimetic Drugs of Piperidine Derivation — CI 395 (Sernyl) and CI 400." *American Journal of Psychiatry* 116(9):843–844.

Liden, D. B.; Lovejoy, F. H.; and Costello, C. E. "Phencyclidine. Nine Cases of Poisoning." *Journal of the American Medical Association* 234:513–516.

Lin, D. C. K.; Fentiman, A. F.; Foltz, R. L.; Forney, R. D.; and Sunshine, I. "Quantification of Phencyclidine in Body Fluids by

Gas Chromatography-Chemical Ionization Mass Spectrometry and Identification of Two Metabolites." *Biomedical Mass Spectrometry* 2:206–215.

Lin, D. C. K.; Foltz, R. L.; Done, A. K.; Aronow, R.; Arcinue, E.; and Miceli, J. N. "Mass Spectrometric Analysis of Phencyclidine in Body Fluids of Intoxicated Patients." In A. P. DeLeenheer and R. R. Roncucci, eds., *Quantitative Mass Spectrometry in Life Sciences,* Amsterdam: Elsevier, 1977, pp. 121–129.

Lindgren, J. E.; Hammer, C. G.; Hessling, R.; and Holmstedt, B. "The Chemical Identity of Hog — A New Hallucinogen." *American Journal of Pharmacy* 141:86–90.

Luby, E. D.; Cohen, B. D.; Rosenbaum, G.; Gottlieb, J. S.; and Kelley, R. "Study of a New Schizophrenamimetic Drug — Sernyl." *Archives of Neurology and Psychiatry* 81:363–369.

Luisada, P. V. "Clinical Experience with Phencyclidine Psychoses." In R. C. Peterson and R. C. Stillman, eds., *Phencyclidine Abuse: An Appraisal.* NIDA Monograph No. 21, U.S. Department of Health, Education, and Welfare No. (ADM) 78-728. Washington, D.C.: U.S. Government Printing Office, 1978.

Luisada, P. V., and Brown, B. L. "Clinical Management of the Phencyclidine Psychosis." *Clinical Toxicology* 9(4):539–545.

Luisada, P. V., and Reddick, C. "An Epidemic of Drug-Induced 'Schizophrenia.' " Paper presented at the 128th annual meeting of the American Psychiatric Association, Anaheim, Calif., May 1975.

Lundberg, G. D.; Gupta, R. C.; and Montgomery, S. H. "Phencyclidine: Patterns Seen in Street Drug Analysis." *Clinical Toxicology* 9(4):503–511.

Lundy, P.; Colhoun, E. H.; and Gowdey, C. W. "Pressor Responses of Ketamine and Circulating Biogenic Amines." *Nature* 241:80–82.

MacLeod, W. D.; Green, D. E.; and Seet, E. "Automated Analysis of Phencyclidine in Urine by Probability Based Matching GC/MS." *Clinical Toxicology* 9(4):561–572.

Marshman, J. A.; Ramsay, M. P.; and Sellers, E. M. "Quantification of Phencyclidine in Biological Fluids and Application to

Human Overdose." *Toxicology and Applied Pharmacology* 35:129–136.

Meibach, R. C.; Glick, S. D.; Cox, R.; and Maayani, S. "Localization of Phencyclidine-Induced Changes in Brain Energy Metabolism." *Nature* 282:625–626.

Meltzer, H. Y. "Effects of Phencyclidine and Restraint at 2°C on Rat Plasma Creatine Phosphokinase Activity." *Research Communications in Chemical Pathology and Pharmacology* 5:117–127.

Meltzer, H. Y. "Muscle Toxicity Produced by Phencyclidine and Restraint Stress." *Research Communications in Chemical Pathology and Pharmacology* 3:369–383.

Meltzer, H. Y.; Fessler, M. S.; Simonovic, M.; and Sturgeon, D. "PCP: Neurochemistry, Treatment, and More." *American Journal of Psychiatry* 136(2):235.

Meltzer, H. Y.; Holzman, P. S.; Hassan, S. Z.; and Guschwan, A. "Effects of Phencyclidine and Stress on Plasma Creatine Phosphokinase (CPK) and Aldolase Activities in Man." *Psychopharmacologia* 26:44–53.

Meyer, J. S.; Greifenstein, F.; and Devault, M. "A New Drug Causing Symptoms of Sensory Deprivation." *Journal of Nervous and Mental Disease* 129:54–61.

Meyers, F. H.; Rose, J. A.; and Smith, D. E. "Incidents Involving the Haight-Ashbury Population and Some Uncommonly Used Drugs." *Journal of Psychedelic Drugs* 1:139–146.

Millo, S., and Chari-Bitron, A. "Effect of Phencyclidine on Oxygen Consumption of Rat Brain Mitochondria in Vitro and in Vivo." *Biochemical Pharmacology* 22:1661–1665.

Morgenstern, F. S.; Beech, H. R.; and Davies, B. M. "An Investigation of Drug Induced Sensory Disturbances." *Psychopharmacologia* 3:193–201.

Muir, B. J.; Evans, J.; and Mulcahy, J. J. "Sernyl Analgesia for Children's Burn Dressings." *British Journal of Anaesthesiology* 33:51–53.

Munch, J. C. "Phencyclidine: Pharmacology and Toxicology." *Bulletin on Narcotics* 26(4):131–133.

Murray, T. F., and Craighill, A. L. "Interactions between Delta 9-Tetrahydrocarbonal and Phencyclidine in Rats and Mice." *Proceedings of the Western Pharmacological Society* 19:362–368.

Neubauer, H.; Sundland, D. M.; and Gershon, S. "Sernyl, Ditran, and Their Antagonists: Succinate and THA." *International Journal of Neuropsychiatry* 2:216–222.

Ober, R. E.; Gwynn, G. W.; McCarthy, D. A.; and Glazko, A. J. "Metabolism of 1-(1-Phenylcyclohexyl) piperidine (Sernyl)." *Federation Proceedings* 22(2), part 1:539–551.

Overton, D. A. "A Comparison of the Discriminable CNS Effects of Ketamine, Phencyclidine and Pentobarbital." *Archives Internationales de Pharmacodynamie et de Therapie* 215:180–189.

Paster, Z.; Maayani, S.; Weinstein, H.; and Sokolovsky, M. "Cholinolytic Action of Phencyclidine Derivatives." *European Journal of Pharmacology* 25:270–274.

Pearce, D. S. "Detection and Quantitation of Phencyclidine in Blood by Use of (2H5) Phencyclidine and Select Ion Monitoring Applied to Non-fatal Cases of Phencyclidine Intoxication." *Clinical Chemistry* 22(10):1623–1626.

Pender, J. W. "Dissociative Anesthesia." *Journal of the American Medical Association* 215:1126–1130.

Perry, D. C. "PCP Revisited." *PharmChem Foundation Newsletter* 4(9):1–7.

Petsonk, C. A., and McAlister, A. L. "Angel Dust: An Overview of Abuse Patterns and Prevention Strategies." *The Journal of School Health* 49(10):565–568.

Pickens, R.; Thompson, T.; and Muchow, D. C. "Cannabis and Phencyclidine Self-Administration by Animals." In L. Goldberg and F. Hoffmeister, eds., *Psychic Dependence. Bayer-Symposium IV.* New York: Springer-Verlag, 1973, pp. 78–86.

Pinchasi, I.; Maayani, S.; and Sokolovsky, M. "On the Interactions of Drugs with the Cholingergic Nervous System. III Tolerance to Phencyclidine Derivatives: In Vivo and in Vitro Studies." *Biochemical Pharmacology* 26:1671.

Pollard, J. C.; Bakker, C.; Uhr, L.; and Feuerfile, D. F. "Controlled Sensory Input: A Note on the Technique of Drug Evaluation with a Preliminary Report on a Comparative Study of Sernyl, Psilocybin, and LSD-25." *Comprehensive Psychiatry* 1:377–380.

Pryor, G. T., and Howd, R. A. "Effects of Chronic Treatment with Morphine, Methadone, and LAAM on the Response to Phencyclidine in Rats." In Louis S. Harris, ed., *Problems of Drug Dependence 1979,* Proceedings of the 41st Annual Scientific Meeting, The Committee on Problems of Drug Dependence, Inc. NIDA Monograph No. 27, U.S. Department of Health, Education, and Welfare No. (ADM) 80-901. Washington, D.C.: U.S. Government Printing Office, 1980.

Rainey, J. M., and Crowder, M. K. "Ketamine or Phencyclidine." *Journal of the American Medical Association* 230:824.

Rainey, J. M., and Crowder, M. K. "More on 'Angel Dust.' " *American Journal of Psychiatry* 132:879.

Rainey, J. M., and Crowder, M. K. "Prevalence of Phencyclidine in Street Drug Preparations." *The New England Journal of Medicine* 290:466–467.

Reed, A., and Kane, A. W. "Phencyclidine (PCP): Another Illicit Psychedelic Drug." *Journal of Psychedelic Drugs* 5:8–12.

Reynolds, P. C. "Clinical and Forensic Experiences with Phencyclidine." *Clinical Toxicology* 9(4):547–552.

Riddoch, M. E. "Evaluation of Phencyclidine (CI-395) for Premedication of Children." *Anaesthesia* 17:419–421.

Rodin, E. A.; Luby, E. D.; and Meyer, J. S. "Electroencephalographic Findings Associated with Sernyl Infusion." *Electroencephalography and Clinical Neurophysiology* 11:796–798.

Roppolo, J. R.; Werner, G.; Whitsel, B. L.; Dreyer, D. A.; and Petrucelli, L. M. "Phencyclidine Action on Neural Mechanisms of Somesthesis." *Neuropharmacology* 12:417–431.

Rosen, A. "Case Report: Symptomatic Mania and Phencyclidine Abuse." *American Journal of Psychiatry* 136(1):118–119.

Rosenbaum, G.; Cohen, B. D.; Luby, E. D.; Gottlieb, J. S.; and

Yelen, D. "Comparison of Sernyl with Other Drugs: Simulation **153** of Schizophrenia Performance with Sernyl, LSD-25, and Amobarbital (Amytal) Sodium I. Attention, Motor Function and Proprioception." *Archives of General Psychiatry* 1:651–656.

Russ, C., and Wong, D. "Diagnosis and Treatment of the Phencyclidine Psychosis: Clinical Considerations." *Journal of Psychedelic Drugs* 11(4):277–282.

Ruwe, D. J. "Preparation of Phencyclidine for the Illicit Market." *Veterinary and Human Toxicology* 21(2):100–101.

Shaffer, L. L. "Ketamine." *Journal of the American Medical Association* 229:763.

Sher, M. D. "Phencyclidine Induced Psychosis and the Insanity Defense." *Criminal Defense* 4(4):5–10.

Shick, J. F. "Epidemiology of Multiple Drug Use with Special Reference to Phencyclidine." In R. C. Peterson and R. C. Stillman, eds., *Phencyclidine Abuse: An Appraisal.* NIDA Monograph No. 21, U.S. Department of Health, Education, and Welfare No. (ADM) 78-728. Washington, D.C.: U.S. Government Printing Office, 1978.

Shulgin, A. T., and MacLean, D. "Illicit Synthesis of Phencyclidine (PCP) and Several of Its Analogues." *Clinical Toxicology* 9(4):553–560.

Simonds, J. F., and Kashani, J. "Phencyclidine Use in Delinquent Males Committed to a Training School." *Adolescence* 14(56):721–725.

Smith, R. C.; Meltzer, H. Y.; Arora, R. C.; and Davis, J. M. "Effects of Phencyclidine on $^3$H-Catecholamine and $^3$H-Serotonin Uptake in Synaptosomal Preparations from Rat Brain." *Biochemical Pharmacology* 26:1435–1439.

Smith, R. C.; Meltzer, H. Y.; Dekirmenjian, H.; and Davis, J. M. "Effects of Phencyclidine on Biogenic Amines in Rat Brain." *Neurosic Abstracts* 1:468.

Soine, W. H.; Vincek, W. C.; and Agee, D. T. "Phencyclidine Contaminant Generates Cyanide." *New England Journal of Medicine* 301(8):438.

**154**

Stein, J. I. "Phencyclidine Induced Psychosis. The Need to Avoid Unnecessary Sensory Influx." *Military Medicine* 138:590–591.

Stockard, J. J.; Werner, S. S.; Aalbers, J. A.; and Chiappa, K. H. "Electroencephalographic Findings in Phencyclidine Intoxication." *Archives of Neurology* 33:200–203.

Taube, H. D.; Montel, H.; Haw, G.; and Starke, K. "Phencyclidine and Ketamine: Comparison with the Effect of Cocaine on the Nonadrenergic Neurons of the Rat Brain Cortex." *Nauyn-Schneideberg's Archives of Pharmacology* 291:47–54.

Thompson, T. N. "Malignant Hyperthermia from PCP." *Journal of Clinical Psychiatry* 40(7):327.

Tong, T. G.; Beowitz, N. L.; Becker, C. E.; Fornia, P. J.; and Boerner, U. "Phencyclidine Poisoning." *Journal of the American Medical Association* 234:512–513.

Tonge, S. R. "Variation of 5-Hydroxytryptamine Metabolism in the Rat: Effects on the Neurochemical Response of Phencyclidine." *Journal of Pharmacy and Pharmacology* 23:71.

Tonge, S. R., and Leonard, B. E. "Interaction of Phencyclidine with Drugs Affecting Noradrenaline Metabolism in the Rat Brain." *Psychopharmacologia* 23:86–90.

Tonge, S. R., and Leonard, B. E. "Partial Antagonism of the Behavioral and Neurochemical Effects of Phencyclidine by Drugs Affecting Monoamine Metabolism." *Psychopharmacologia* 24:516–520.

Tonge, S. R., and Leonard, B. E. "Variation in Hydroxytryptamine Metabolism in the Rat: Effects on the Neurochemical Response to Phencyclidine." *Journal of Pharmacy and Pharmacology* 23:711–712.

Traber, D. L.; Wilson, R. D.; and Priano, L. L. "Differentiation of the Cardiovascular Effects of CI-581." *Anesthesia and Analgesia, Current Researches* 47(6):769–778.

Tweed, W. A.; Minuck, M.; and Mymin, D. "Circulatory Responses to Ketamine Anesthesia." *Anesthesiology* 37(6):613–619.

Vincent, J. P.; Cavey, K.; Kamenka, J. M.; Geneste, P.; and Lazdunski, M. "Interaction of Phencyclidines with the Muscarinic and Opiate Receptors in the Central Nervous System." *Brain Research* 152:176–182.

Wilson, A. E., and Domino, E. F. "Plasma Phencyclidine Pharmacokinetics in Dog and Monkey Using a Gas Chromatography Selected Ion Monitoring Assay." *Biomedical Mass Spectrometry* 5(2):112–116.

**155**

# 156    Film List

Film Tree Distributors
P.O. Box 84346
Los Angeles, California 90073

☐    The PCP Story (Art–Co Productions)
☐    Angel Dust/PCP (CBS 60 Minutes)
☐    PCP Laboratory Seizure and Take Down:
Peace Officer and Firefighter Survival

Media Five
3211 Cahuenga Blvd.
West Hollywood, California 90063

☐    Angel Death

Chuck Wintner Productions
2330 Sixth Street, Suite 2
Santa Monica, California 90405

☐    Angel Dust

# PCP Abuse Training Outline

| Content | Human Service Providers | | | | |
|---|:---:|:---:|:---:|:---:|:---:|
| | Criminal Justice | Emergency Medicine | Mental Health | Drug Abuse Treatment | Education |
| I. Overview of PCP and Polydrug Abuse | | | | | |
|   A. Orientation to Polydrug Abuse | √ | √ | √ | √ | √ |
|     1. The History of Polydrug Abuse | | | | | |
|       a. Early use of psychoactive substances | | | | | |
|       b. Medical–social issues | | | | | |
|       c. Current patterns of polydrug abuse | | | | | |
|       d. Future trends? | | | | | |
|     2. How Drugs Affect Behavior | | | | | |
|       a. The person | | | | | |
|       b. The environment | | | | | |
|       c. Expectations | | | | | |
|       d. Pharmacokinetics, principles of drug action | | | | | |
|     3. The Psychological Aspects of Polydrug Abuse | | | | | |
|       a. Basic human needs | | | | | |
|       b. Profiles of polydrug abusers | | | | | |
|       c. Drugs: both symptom and cause | | | | | |
|     4. The Sociological Aspects of Polydrug Abuse | | | | | |
|       a. Family systems | | | | | |
|       b. Peer influence | | | | | |
|       c. Culture change | | | | | |
|     5. The Impact of Media on Polydrug Abuse | | | | | |
|       a. Advertising and persuasion | | | | | |
|       b. Alternatives to reducing drug abuse | | | | | |

| Content | Criminal Justice | Emergency Medicine | Mental Health | Drug Abuse Treatment | Education |
|---|:-:|:-:|:-:|:-:|:-:|
| **B. Overview of the PCP Problem** | √ | √ | √ | √ | √ |
|   1. The Evolution of PCP Abuse | | | | | |
|     a. A new class of drugs | | | | | |
|     b. Clinical studies in animals | | | | | |
|     c. Experimental use on humans | | | | | |
|     d. The illicit use of PCP | | | | | |
|       (1) The PCP experience | | | | | |
|       (2) PCP and sexuality | | | | | |
|   2. Epidemiology of PCP Abuse | | | | | |
|     a. Patterns of abuse | | | | | |
|     b. Major areas of abuse | | | | | |
|     c. Prevalence of abuse | | | | | |
|     d. Characteristics of PCPers | | | | | |
|   3. Street Pharmacology | | | | | |
|     a. Forms | | | | | |
|     b. Packaging | | | | | |
|     c. Modes of administration | | | | | |
|     d. Amount of PCP by forms used | | | | | |
|   4. The Psychology of the PCPer | | | | | |
|     a. Profile | | | | | |
|     b. Social relationships | | | | | |
|     c. Music | | | | | |
|     d. Risk-taking behavior | | | | | |
|     e. Longevity | | | | | |

Human Service Providers

| Content | Human Service Providers | | | | |
|---|---|---|---|---|---|
| | Criminal Justice | Emergency Medicine | Mental Health | Drug Abuse Treatment | Education |
| 5. Impact of PCP on the Community | | | | | |
|    a. Cost to the PCPer | | | | | |
|    b. Cost to others | | | | | |
| 6. Unanswered Questions | | | | | |
|    a. PCP and brain damage | | | | | |
|    b. Analogs | | | | | |
|    c. Metabolites | | | | | |
| II. Recognizing and Managing the PCPer | | | | | |
| A. Guidelines for Recognizing the PCPer | | | | | |
| 1. The Intoxicated State | √ | √ | √ | √ | √ |
|    a. Observable effects | | | | | |
|    b. Clinical interpretations | | | | | |
| 2. Presumptive Testing | √ | | | | |
| 3. Levels of Intoxication | √ | √ | √ | √ | √ |
|    a. Confusional state | | | | | |
|    b. Agitated state | | | | | |
|    c. Comatose state | | | | | |
| 4. Types of PCPers | √ | √ | √ | √ | √ |
|    a. Experimental | | | | | |
|    b. Recreational | | | | | |
|    c. Chronic | | | | | |

| Content | Criminal Justice | Emergency Medicine | Mental Health | Drug Abuse Treatment | Education |
|---|:-:|:-:|:-:|:-:|:-:|
| 5. Emergency Medical Diagnosis | | ✓ | ✓ | | |
|    a. Toxicological screening | | | | | |
|    b. Differential diagnoses | | | | | |
|    c. Documentation of PCP intoxication and related findings | | | | | |
| B. Guidelines for Managing PCP Abuse | | | | | |
| 1. General Guidelines for Managing the PCPer | ✓ | ✓ | ✓ | ✓ | ✓ |
| 2. Emergency Medical Treatment | | ✓ | ✓ | ✓ | |
|    a. Confusional state | | | | | |
|    b. Agitated state | | | | | |
|    c. Comatose state | | | | | |
|    d. Ion trapping– acidification procedure | | | | | |
|    e. Hospital discharge and referral | | | | | |
| 3. Drug Counseling and Treatment Services | | ✓ | ✓ | ✓ | |
|    a. Prolonged psychosis | | | | | |
|      (1) In-patients | | | | | |
|        (a) Orientation | | | | | |
|        (b) Integration | | | | | |
|        (c) Habilitation | | | | | |
|      (2) Outpatients | | | | | |
|      (3) Staffing | | | | | |
|      (4) Setting | | | | | |
|      (5) Procedures | | | | | |

Human Service Providers

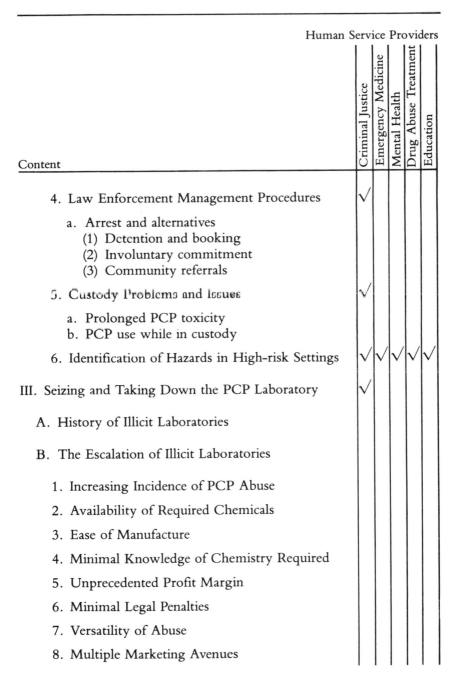

| Content | Human Service Providers | | | | |
|---|---|---|---|---|---|
| | Criminal Justice | Emergency Medicine | Mental Health | Drug Abuse Treatment | Education |
| 4. Law Enforcement Management Procedures | √ | | | | |
|    a. Arrest and alternatives | | | | | |
|      (1) Detention and booking | | | | | |
|      (2) Involuntary commitment | | | | | |
|      (3) Community referrals | | | | | |
| 5. Custody Problems and Issues | √ | | | | |
|    a. Prolonged PCP toxicity | | | | | |
|    b. PCP use while in custody | | | | | |
| 6. Identification of Hazards in High-risk Settings | √ | √ | √ | √ | √ |
| III. Seizing and Taking Down the PCP Laboratory | √ | | | | |
|   A. History of Illicit Laboratories | | | | | |
|   B. The Escalation of Illicit Laboratories | | | | | |
|     1. Increasing Incidence of PCP Abuse | | | | | |
|     2. Availability of Required Chemicals | | | | | |
|     3. Ease of Manufacture | | | | | |
|     4. Minimal Knowledge of Chemistry Required | | | | | |
|     5. Unprecedented Profit Margin | | | | | |
|     6. Minimal Legal Penalties | | | | | |
|     7. Versatility of Abuse | | | | | |
|     8. Multiple Marketing Avenues | | | | | |

| Content | Human Service Providers | | | | |
|---|---|---|---|---|---|
| | Criminal Justice | Emergency Medicine | Mental Health | Drug Abuse Treatment | Education |
| C. Production of Analogs | | | | | |
| D. Variability of Laboratory Settings | | | | | |
| E. Illicit PCP Manufacture and the Law | | | | | |
| F. Detection of Illicit Phencyclidine Laboratories | | | | | |
| 1. Chemical Company Surveillance | | | | | |
| 2. Department of Justice Records | | | | | |
| 3. Drug Enforcement | | | | | |
| 4. Chemical Odors | | | | | |
| 5. Explosions and/or Fires | | | | | |
| 6. Observations and Citizen Reports | | | | | |
| 7. Informant Reports | | | | | |
| 8. Common Indicators of Illicit Laboratory Sites | | | | | |
| G. Manufacture of the Phencyclidines | | | | | |
| 1. Chemical Identification | | | | | |
| 2. Equipment Identification | | | | | |
| 3. Toxicity of Chemicals and Major Reactions | | | | | |
| 4. Other Dangers | | | | | |

| Content | Human Service Providers | | | | |
|---|---|---|---|---|---|
| | Criminal Justice | Emergency Medicine | Mental Health | Drug Abuse Treatment | Education |
| H. Investigative Issues | | | | | |
|   1. Surveillance | | | | | |
|   2. Personnel Requirements | | | | | |
|   3. Equipment Requirements | | | | | |
| I. Laboratory Search, Seizure, and Take Down | | | | | |
|   1. Personnel Requirements | | | | | |
|   2. Containment | | | | | |
|   3. Safety Guidelines | | | | | |
|   4. Equipment Requirements | | | | | |
|   5. Legal Authority | | | | | |
|     a. Warrants | | | | | |
|     b. Case law | | | | | |
| J. Evidence Collection, Transport, Preservation, Storage, and Disposal | | | | | |
|   1. Site Photography | | | | | |
|   2. Latent Prints | | | | | |
|   3. Sample Related Evidence Collection | | | | | |
|   4. Disposal of Excessive Chemicals | | | | | |
|     a. Court order | | | | | |
|     b. Class A dump permit | | | | | |

| Content | Criminal Justice | Emergency Medicine | Mental Health | Drug Abuse Treatment | Education |
|---|---|---|---|---|---|
| Human Service Providers | | | | | |
| c. Personnel requirements | | | | | |
| d. Vehicle code requirements | | | | | |
| 5. Storage of Evidence | | | | | |
| a. Space ventilation, equipment requirements, and handling procedure | | | | | |
| b. Toxicity of chemicals in evidence | | | | | |
| c. Dangers | | | | | |
| IV. Litigating PCP-Related Offenses | √ | √ | √ | | |
| A. PCP and the Law | | (Expert Witnesses) | | | |
| 1. Under the Influence and Personal Use | | | | | |
| 2. Possession and Sale | | | | | |
| 3. Manufacturing | | | | | |
| 4. Federal Law | | | | | |
| 5. Case Law | | | | | |
| 6. Civil Liability | | | | | |
| B. Legal Implications of PCP-Related Acts | | | | | |
| 1. Driving Under the Influence | | | | | |
| 2. Robbery and Burglary | | | | | |
| 3. Arson | | | | | |
| 4. Rape | | | | | |

| | Human Service Providers | | | | |
|---|---|---|---|---|---|
| Content | Criminal Justice | Emergency Medicine | Mental Health | Drug Abuse Treatment | Education |
| 5. Child Endangering | | | | | |
| 6. Homicide | | | | | |
| 7. Others | | | | | |
| C. PCP, Diminished Capacity, and Insanity | | | | | |
| 1. Homicide | | | | | |
| a. First degree murder and felony murder | | | | | |
| b. Second degree murder | | | | | |
| c. Manslaughter | | | | | |
| 2. Prerequisites to Interrogation | | | | | |
| 3. Diminished Capacity | | | | | |
| 4. Insanity | | | | | |
| 5. Differentiation | | | | | |
| D. PCP Case Preparation | | | | | |
| 1. Writing the Report | | | | | |
| 2. Preparing Evidence | | | | | |
| a. Collection | | | | | |
| b. Preservation | | | | | |
| c. Documentation and verification | | | | | |
| d. Booking | | | | | |

| Content | Criminal Justice | Emergency Medicine | Mental Health | Drug Abuse Treatment | Education |
|---|---|---|---|---|---|
| | | | Human Service Providers | | |
| 3. Preparing for Testifying | | | | | |
|    a. Toxicology | | | | | |
|    b. Medical findings | | | | | |
|    c. Defendants' statements | | | | | |
|    d. Statements of witnesses | | | | | |
|    e. Conduct and condition of suspect while in custody | | | | | |
| E. Requirements of the Testifying Officer | | | | | |
|    1. Verify PCP Intoxication | | | | | |
|    2. Describe Effects of PCP | | | | | |
|    3. Others | | | | | |
| V. Public Awareness and Prevention | √ | | √ | √ | √ |
| A. Factors Related to Public Awareness and Prevention | | | | | |
|    1. Nature and Extent of PCP Abuse in the Community | | | | | |
|    2. Community Resources | | | | | |
|    3. Interagency Cooperation | | | | | |
|    4. Existing Public Awareness and Prevention Activities | | | | | |
|    5. Need for Community Action Planning | | | | | |
| B. Principles of Prevention | | | | | |

| Content | Human Service Providers | | | | |
|---|---|---|---|---|---|
| | Criminal Justice | Emergency Medicine | Mental Health | Drug Abuse Treatment | Education |
| C. Community Network Building | | | | | |
|   1. The Network Model | | | | | |
|   2. Community Action Process | | | | | |
|   3. Network Components | | | | | |
|     a. Demand for services | | | | | |
|     b. Resources | | | | | |
|     c. Task force committee | | | | | |
|     d. Community awareness | | | | | |
|     e. Interagency advisory council | | | | | |
| D. Multicultural Issues | | | | | |
|   1. Ethnic | | | | | |
|   2. Sex | | | | | |
|   3. Other Human Service Providers | | | | | |
| E. Public Awareness and Prevention Strategies | | | | | |
|   1. Media | | | | | |
|     a. Radio | | | | | |
|     b. Television | | | | | |
|     c. Print | | | | | |
|   2. Schools | | | | | |
|   3. Voluntary and Community Service Programs | | | | | |
|   4. Other | | | | | |